D1252670

DATE DUE / DATE DE

The Canadian

Dental

Office

Administrator

The Canadian
Dental
Office
Administrator

310101
AES-3617

Sandie Baillargeon
Career Canada College

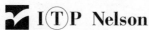

I(T)P Nelson

an International Thomson Publishing company

Toronto • Albany • Bonn • Boston • Cincinnati • Detroit • London • Madrid • Melbourne
Mexico City • New York • Pacific Grove • Paris • San Francisco • Singapore • Tokyo • Washington

I(T)P® International Thomson Publishing

The ITP logo is a trademark under licence
http://www.thomsom.com

Published in 1997 by
I(T)P® Nelson

A division of Thomson Canada Limited
1120 Birchmount Road
Scarborough, Ontario M1K 5G4

http://www.nelson.com

Canadian Cataloguing in Publication Data

Baillargeon, Sandie, 1956-
    The Canadian dental office administrator

Includes index.
ISBN 0-17-606985-2

1. Dental offices - Canada - Management.   I. Title.

RK58.7.C3B34 1997   651'.96176   C96-932501-0

Publisher and Team Leader	Jacqueline Wood
Acquisitions Editor	Jennifer Dewey
Senior Editor	Rosalyn Steiner
Project Editor	Jenny Anttila
Copy Editor	Lynda Chiotti
Senior Production Coordinator	Carol Tong
Art Director	Sylvia Vander Schee
Interior Design	Stephen Boyle
Cover Design	Sylvia Vander Schee
Composition	Anita Macklin

Printed and bound in Canada
1 2 3 4 BBM 00 99 98 97

CONTENTS

Preface   xiii

CHAPTER ONE

THE DENTAL OFFICE ADMINISTRATOR:
THE KEY TO A SUCCESSFUL PRACTICE   1

Dentistry in the 21st Century   1
Administrative Functions   3
   Model Job Description   4
How Do Patients Select A Dental Office?   7
The Dental Office Environment   8
Protecting the Patients   9
Personal Qualities   9
Employment Opportunities   11
Assignment   12

CHAPTER TWO

PATIENT COMMUNICATIONS   13

Applied Psychology   13
   Understanding Patient Behaviour   15
Communication Skills   18
   Qualities of Good Communicators   19
   Barriers to Patient Communications   22
   Practising Communication Skills with New Patients   23
Assignment   23

CHAPTER THREE

DENTAL TERMINOLOGY   24

Word Formation   24
   Word Parts   25
   Numbers   26
   Colours   26
Glossary of Dental Terms   27
Assignment   36

CHAPTER FOUR

TOOTH MORPHOLOGY   38

Parts of the Mouth   38

Types of Teeth   40
Structure of a Tooth   42
The Eruption Cycle of Teeth   42
Tooth Surfaces   44
Assignment   46

CHAPTER FIVE

TOOTH IDENTIFICATION AND NUMBERING SYSTEMS   47

Importance of Tooth Identification   47
International Tooth Numbering System   48
Universal Tooth Numbering System   52
Palmer's Identification System   53
Assignment   56

CHAPTER SIX

UNDERSTANDING THE DENTAL CHART   58

Medical Histories   58
Health Alerts   60
Purposes of the Dental Chart   61
Transferring Patient Records   63
Charting   63
Assignment   67

CHAPTER SEVEN

DENTAL INSURANCE   69

What is Insurance?   69
Eligibility Requirements   70
Assignment of Benefits   71
Capitation Program   71
Preferred Provider Organization   72
Shared Risk   72
Exclusions and Limitations   74
Predetermination of Benefits   75
Coordination of Benefits   76
Understanding the Fee Guide   78
Instructions for Completing Claim Forms   79
Electronic Data Interchange   82
Assignment   83

CHAPTER EIGHT

APPOINTMENT SCHEDULING   86

Key to Productivity   86

The Appointment Book   87
    Selecting an Appointment Book   87
    Factors to Consider   88
Scheduling Appointments   88
    Confirming Appointments   89
Preparing for Appointments   89
    Colour Coding Schedules   91
Cancellation and Short Notice Lists   92
New Patient Procedure   93
Determine and Plan the Ideal Day   93
    Set Goals for Financial Productivity   94
    Double Booking   95
    Emergency versus Urgency   95
    Buffer Zones   96
    Staff Meetings   96
School Holidays   97
Series of Appointments   97
Scheduling Patients with Special Needs   97
Time Management   98
    Late Patients   98
    Continuing Care Appointments   98
    Changing from Manual to Computerized Scheduling   99
Assignment   99

CHAPTER NINE

EFFECTIVE TELEPHONE SKILLS   102

Front Line of Communications   102
    Voice Quality   103
Anatomy of the Telephone Call   105
Emergency versus Urgency   105
Legal Issues   106
Equipment and Technology   106
    Voice Mail   108
    Electronic Mail   108
    The Hold Button   108
Telephone System Management   108
    Collection Calls   109
    Continuing Care Calls   109
    Follow-Up Calls   110
    Angry Calls   110
    Taking Messages   110
    Screening Calls   112
Assignment   113

CHAPTER TEN

RECALL SYSTEMS   114

Continuing Care   114
Patient Attitudes Toward Health Care   115
Why is a Recall System Important to the Patient?   115
Types of Recall Systems   116
    Telephone System   116
    Mail System   117
    Continuous Appointment System   118
    Combination Recall System   119
    Computerized Recall Systems   120
Assignment   121

CHAPTER ELEVEN

ACCOUNTS RECEIVABLE   122

Importance of Financial Control   122
The One Write Bookkeeping System   125
Leaflet Receipts   125
The Ledger Card   127
    Posting Daily Entries   129
The Daysheet   130
    Daily Balancing Procedure   131
    Steps to Balancing   132
Advance Payments   133
Refunds of Credit Balances   133
Bad Debts   133
NSF Cheques   133
Balancing the Accounts Receivable   134
Financial Arrangements   134
    Methods of Payment   135
Collection Procedures   136
    Statements   136
    Collection Letters   136
    Collection Agencies   136
Assignment   140

CHAPTER TWELVE

ACCOUNTS PAYABLE   141

Key Concepts   141
The Disbursements Journal   142
Expense Categories   142
    Description of Expense Categories   143
Writing Cheques   145
    The Petty Cash Fund   147
Bill Payments   149
Inventory Control   149
Assignment   150

CHAPTER THIRTEEN

PAYROLL	151
Payroll Considerations	151
Time Records	152
New Employees	152
Social Insurance Number	153
Employer/Employee Relationship	155
Source Deductions	155
Income Tax	156
Canada Pension Plan	156
Unemployment Insurance	156
Remitting Deductions	158
T4 Slips	160
Vacation Pay	160
Record of Employment	161
Assignment	163

CHAPTER FOURTEEN

BANKING	164
Responsibilities	164
Bank Services	165
Current Accounts	165
Cheques	165
Bank Deposits	169
Payment Options	169
Credit Card Payments	169
Bank Reconciliation	171
Steps to Reconciliation	171
If the Reconciliation Does Not Balance	172
Assignment	173

CHAPTER FIFTEEN

RECORDS MANAGEMENT	175
Importance of Confidentiality	175
Records Protection	176
Retention of Records	177
Release of Information	178
Informed Consent	178
The Clinical Record	178
Medical Histories	182
Financial Records	182
Filing Systems	183
Equipment	183
Equipment Safety	183

Filing   184
Assignment   186

CHAPTER SIXTEEN

PREVENTIVE DENTISTRY AND PATHOLOGY   187

Preventive Dentistry   187
   Healthy Teeth for a Lifetime   188
   Patient Education   188
   Pit and Fissure Sealants   189
Causes of Dental Disease   189
   The Formation of Plaque   190
Nutrition and Oral Health   190
   Fluoride   191
   Toothbrushing Techniques   191
The Recall Appointment   192
Dental Pathology   193
   Gingivitis   193
   Periodontitis   193
   Necrotizing Ulcerative Gingivitis   194
   Glossitis   194
Assignment   195

CHAPTER SEVENTEEN

PHARMACOLOGY   196

Prescription Drugs   196
   The Prescription   197
   Types of Drugs Commonly Prescribed   199
   Routes of Drug Administration   202
Narcotics Control   204
Drug Action   207
Medications Management   208
Premedication Procedures   208
Assignment   211

CHAPTER EIGHTEEN

MARKETING THE DENTAL PRACTICE   212

What Is Marketing?   212
   Product and Price   213
   Location   214
Informed Choices   214
The Role of the Dental Team in Marketing Strategy   215
Patient/Provider Trust   216
The Marketing Plan   217
   Electronic Marketing   218

Specific Marketing Ideas 219
Continuing Education and the Dental Team 220
Assignment 221

CHAPTER NINETEEN

PERSONNEL RELATIONS 223

Office Management 223
Hiring the Right Team Member 224
Guidelines to Hiring 225
Résumés 227
Office Philosophy 227
Office Policies 227
The Staff Meeting 228
The Morning Meeting 229
Delegation of Duties 229
Role Model 230
Problem Solving 231
Staff Incentives 232
Assignment 233

CHAPTER TWENTY

WRITTEN COMMUNICATIONS 234

The Challenge of Communications 234
Methods of Spelling Improvement 235
Dictionary Usage 236
Grammar 236
Sentence Structure 239
Punctuation 241
Letter Styles 246
Assignment 251

CHAPTER TWENTY-ONE

ORGANIZATIONAL TECHNIQUES 253

Procedures and Protocol Manual 253
Master Copies of Forms 255
Chronological Filing System 255
Recall Cards 256
Follow-Up Binder 256
Insurance Code Reference Sheet 257
Setting Goals 257
Assignment 257

CHAPTER TWENTY-TWO

THE JOB SEARCH   258

What Employers Expect   258
    Skills   259
    Attendance and Punctuality   259
Attitude   260
A Systematic Approach to the Job Search   260
    Rejection   260
    Planning the Strategy   261
The Résumé   263
    Functions of the Résumé   263
    The Cover Letter   264
The Interview   265
Concerns of the Potential Employer   267
Salary Negotiations   270
    Follow-Up   270
    Once You Are Hired   271
Assignment   271

CHAPTER TWENTY-THREE

COMPUTERS IN DENTAL OFFICES   272

Computer Literacy   272
What Is a Computer?   273
    Fears Associated with Learning to Use Computers   273
    Needs Analysis   274
    Hardware   275
    Software   279
Patient Information   280
Electronic Data Interchange   282
Ergonomics   283
    Care and Maintenance of Computers   284
    Computer Support   289
Assignment   289

INDEX   290

As dental teams prepare to meet the challenges of the 21st century, they need to assume a wider range of responsibilities even while they face fierce competition in the marketplace. These challenges create a unique opportunity for dental administrators to augment their education and enhance their skill base. *The Canadian Dental Office Administrator* examines the key role dental administrators assume in managing the dental business office.

Dental office administrators are management professionals whose expertise affects the financial productivity, stress level, and overall professional image of the dental practice. They play an important role in today's competitive environment. My primary objective has been to create a balance between theoretical knowledge and practical applications.

This project arose from careful and diligent research in an effort to produce a comprehensive manual with information relevant to Canadian dental office administrators. The text is structured to allow students to build on each successive lesson and to practise the applications discussed. Skills are presented and examined in a logical sequence. Emphasis has been placed on all aspects of dental office management in order to address the concerns of this progressive industry.

The book includes a significant amount of information regarding marketing, patient communications, staff relations, and personal growth topics that will enable the dental office administrator to make a strong contribution to a dental practice while providing an opportunity for developing a fulfilling career.

Each chapter provides a behavioural objective and a list of topics to be addressed. The book has been structured into three sections.

1. The beginning chapters cover the duties and responsibilities of the dental office administrator, including communication skills and the psychological aspects of human interaction.
2. The second section provides a basis of clinical theory in order to understand the language of dentistry. The dental office administrator acts as the liaison between the doctor and the patient, and often must interpret highly technical information into understandable terms for the client.
3. The latter chapters include practical office management skills that are applicable to the daily operation of a progressive dental office. They also address the issues of job searching and computer basics. Since many dental software programs are particular to each office,

it is impossible to include all the information that is available. It is assumed that individual training will be provided in a separate course or on the job.

This text has been designed to become a desktop reference on completion of the related course material.

ACKNOWLEDGMENTS

I wish to express my sincere appreciation to my colleagues who contributed their knowledge and expertise so willingly during the preparation of this book. I would like to thank the following people, who reviewed draft chapters early in the process and provided valuable feedback: S. Gayle Charsley, Cambrian College; Marlene Hamilton, Conestoga College; Jo Szabo, Niagara College; Rosemarie Turton, St. Clair College; Linda Vaessen, Fanshawe College; and Kim Walker, Canadore College. Special appreciation should be given to the students and faculty of Career Canada College who provided me with the inspiration. My thanks also to Dr. Art Tupper, Dr. Gord Davidson, and Dr. John Adams for their support and encouragement, and to my dear friend and colleague Mary Brioux for her loyal friendship and for serving as a role model. In addition, special thank you to Joy Little, Coordinator of the Dental Chairside Assisting Department at Career Canada College and Chair for the Continuing Education Committee, Canadian Dental Assistants Association. Along with her support and friendship, Mrs. Little contributed her clinical expertise and enhanced the technical information contained in this text.

A very special thanks to George Scalia who was instrumental in encouraging the adoption of this project. Great appreciation is given to Jennifer Dewey, Jenny Anttila, and Rosalyn Steiner for their on-going support, expertise, and patience.

Special appreciation is given to the following provincial association members for their helpful feedback from the inception to the completion of the manuscript: Louise Mabey, President of the Canadian Dental Assistants Association; Joyce Acheson and Aldine Walling, The Alberta Dental Assistants Association; Susan Anholt, The Saskatchewan Dental Assistants' Association; Marlene Robinson, The College of Dental Surgeons of British Columbia.

In particular I would like to thank my family for their constant motivation and support, and for understanding my temporary preoccupation and absence from their daily lives. Finally, my appreciation to my close friends and colleagues for their support.

SANDIE BAILLARGEON

To the Canadian Dental Office Administrator

and to Tim and Sabrina for their

constant love and support

CHAPTER ONE

The Dental Office Administrator: The Key to a Successful Practice

OBJECTIVE

At the end of this chapter, the student will be able to identify and describe the following: duties and responsibilities of a dental office administrator, some universal concerns of dentists, methods for controlling stress while increasing productivity, factors influencing how patients select a dental office, and employment opportunities.

TOPICS

- the dental team
- model job description
- personal qualities of the dental office administrator
- how patients select a dental office
- common concerns of dental professionals

DENTISTRY IN THE 21ST CENTURY

Dentistry, like most industries, has gone through many changes that reflect trends in the economy, rapid technological development, and fierce competition. Dental practitioners are compelled to operate their practices as effectively as possible while maintaining cost control. The traditional approach of specializing in one particular area is changing in response to a demanding workplace. Now most dental professionals must know a variety of job skills in order to be successful.

Dentists seek potential employees who have a variety of skills that are applicable to several aspects of practice management. To maintain their own competitive edge, dentists need employees who have a thorough understanding of the day-to-day operations of the *business* of dentistry.

For example, the formula for an ideal dental office administrator may look something like this:

A dental assistant + reception skills + computer skills (operations and maintenance) + business knowledge + strong interpersonal skills + marketing expertise = a well-qualified dental office administrator.

The dictionary defines "team" as "a number of persons associated in work or activity." To work together as a team, each member of the dental office must learn as much as possible about every aspect of practice administration to complement the clinical skills of the service providers.

Dentists have come to realize the importance of delegating management responsibilities to their office administrators. It is no longer feasible to hire an employee who requires extensive training. A candidate for employment should be highly skilled and motivated. In addition, the candidate should be prepared to make a strong contribution to the success of the dental practice immediately.

Dentistry is a health care profession; however, it is also a business. Canadian dentists spend most of their educational years becoming excellent diagnosticians and perfecting their clinical skills. Comparatively little educational time is used to learn practice management skills.

A new dentist faces several challenges: where to draw new patients from, how to hire staff, how much to pay staff, how to deal with personnel problems, and how to build and maintain a profitable business. These are only some of the universal concerns that the dentist faces in starting and operating a successful practice. Fierce competition within the dental community and advertising or marketing limitations add further pressure to the new dentist.

Many Canadian dentists operate their practices with overhead costs of 60 percent or greater of total monthly fees charged. Therefore, even when the practice has been established, it is a continuous challenge to keep it viable.

The dental office administrator provides a crucial link in communication between the patient, the dentist, and the staff, as well as the community. Dentists will delegate the business responsibilities to their staff and rely on the administrator to be the binding force. This allows dentists to do what they do best, practise the art of dentistry.

ADMINISTRATIVE FUNCTIONS

The dental office administrator is the key to the successful practice. The first face that the patient sees in the office or the first voice over the telephone is that of the administrator.

The office administrator manages the stress level in the office as well as the financial productivity of the practice. These tasks require a person who is committed to the success of the practice, who is highly motivated and well organized and who can provide patients with comfort.

Creative appointment scheduling helps the administrator to increase financial productivity while controlling stress. Communication with the clinical staff is essential. It is important to understand shared concerns and to assist in problem resolution whenever possible. This promotes a sense of cooperation throughout the office.

Educating patients about the financial policies of the office helps them to understand and cooperate with payment. Patients should feel that they have a choice of payment options, yet the administrator must retain control over the accounts receivable.

A dental office administrator will set daily production goals and be aware of the costs of keeping the practice viable. Monitoring progress toward these goals will help to keep the practice on track.

Using an efficient recall system and following through with treatment plans are effective ways of controlling the financial productivity of a practice and promoting repeat business. The dental office administrator should know what affects patient behaviour and understand why patients select a particular dental office.

In summary, the dental office administrator should display a professional and mature attitude and should be well organized, committed to the success of the practice, and a team player. Maintaining a state of good health and personal happiness also helps to project an image of overall wellness. Above all, the administrator should exhibit a positive outlook. These personal attributes reflect the professional image of the office.

Model Job Description

The dental office administrator will conduct and coordinate the daily activities necessary to delivery of optimal dental health care. This person will manage all aspects of patient scheduling and flow, the clinical and financial records of the business, inventory, patient communications, and recall systems.

Knowledge, Skills, and Abilities

1. Minimum education level of a related diploma or the equivalent in work experience and continuing education.
2. Knowledge of dental terminology, dental morphology, dental insurance, preventive dentistry, accounts receivable, accounts payable, payroll, and records management.
3. Knowledge of the Canadian Dental Association Code of Ethics.
4. Knowledge of personnel relations and employment standards.
5. Excellent written and oral communications skills, including English usage, grammar, punctuation, and style.
6. Ability to work independently with minimal supervision.
7. Ability to work under pressure with time constraints.
8. Ability to concentrate.
9. Ability to use interpersonal skills effectively to build and maintain cooperative working relationships.
10. Provincial Certification status or business credentials preferred.

Job Responsibilities and Performance Standards

1. *Patient Management*

   - greet patients, schedule appointments
   - educate patients regarding office policies, including cancellation and financial policy
   - provide patients with comfort

2. *Appointment Book Control*

   - schedule creatively to maximize production and minimize stress
   - create and maintain effective follow-up procedures
   - maintain a "short notice" list
   - create a reminder system
   - prepare colour coded schedules for each treatment room
   - maintain control of the appointment book
   - maintain daily patient flow
   - develop and administer cancellation policy

3. *Recall System*

   - develop and maintain an effective system to recall patients for follow-up care and preventive appointments
   - encourage and promote patient loyalty and referrals

4. *Patient Records*

   - complete and maintain a comprehensive clinical and financial record for each patient
   - purge and condition charts regularly
   - protect the confidential nature of all records, especially the clinical records of the patient
   - file and store charts properly
   - maintain records of preventive care

5. *Dental Insurance*

   - complete insurance forms, predeterminations
   - follow up insurance claims
   - assist patients to understand their insurance programs
   - apply the appropriate fee guide codes and tooth identification codes

6. *Telephone Tasks*

   - manage all incoming and outgoing telephone calls
   - practise courteous and professional telephone techniques
   - take messages
   - make collection calls
   - schedule appointments
   - screen calls to the dentist
   - determine the difference between an "urgency" and an "emergency"

7. *Correspondence*

   - apply excellent written communication skills including correct grammar, punctuation, and style to all office correspondence
   - project a professional image on all forms of written communication

8. *Financial Records*

- manage the accounts receivable and accounts payable
- balance the daily and monthly accounts receivable and payable records
- maintain daily and monthly production records
- prepare monthly statements for the dentist
- prepare monthly statements to patients
- execute collection procedures for negligent accounts, including letters and calls

9. *Inventory*

- verify invoices and statements
- maintain a subject filing system
- deal with salespeople
- develop and implement an equipment maintenance program

10. *Banking Procedures*

- prepare bank deposits
- reconcile bank statements
- write cheques

11. *Payroll*

- maintain payroll administration records
- understand and implement a policy for employee standards
- follow Revenue Canada guidelines and procedures for payroll administration, including submission of payroll deductions
- prepare the *Record of Employment* for employees who have left the practice
- maintain a supply of the forms required
- provide support and information to staff members

12. *Staff Coordination*

- practise conflict resolution and problem solving
- listen and respond to concerns of staff and patients
- offer support to staff and patients as needed
- organize the agenda for staff meetings
- act as a role model

13. *Marketing*

- create, coordinate, and implement an internal marketing program
- involve all members of the dental team in the creative process of marketing dental services
- establish an office philosophy and image
- incorporate "point-of-sale" marketing techniques into daily operations

14. *Patient Consultations*

- discuss treatment plans, and make financial arrangements in accordance with the office financial policy
- be sensitive to the needs of the patient

15. *Personal Growth*

- maintain professional standards through continued education and upgrading of skills
- participate, communicate, and cooperate with the dentist, staff, and patients on all appropriate levels

The remaining chapters of this book will address each of these job responsibilities and provide guidelines to enhance the development of job skills and performance objectives.

HOW DO PATIENTS SELECT A DENTAL OFFICE?

A patient's selection of a dental office is based on many factors. The most important source of new patients is personal referrals. A patient who has a positive experience at a dental office will refer friends, relatives, and others. If a patient has a negative experience, word spreads quickly throughout the community. One who has a positive experience may tell three people, but someone who has a negative experience is likely to tell 11 people.

A patient is seldom able to select a dental office based entirely on knowledge of the dentist's clinical ability. The decision is usually based on a combination of factors such as location, office hours, office cleanliness, and the friendliness of the staff. Often a patient will visit the office to judge the cleanliness of the surroundings, evaluate how comfortable he or she feels with the staff, and form a first impression of the office.

Very few people evaluate dental services based on the fees only. In fact, most people will pay the appropriate fees willingly if they feel that they and their families are being well cared for and their needs are being met. Most patients are willing to pay for a high quality service if they feel that the service is worth it.

The first impression that the patient receives is usually the most lasting. The dental office administrator is responsible for creating and projecting a positive first impression. This is one of the most important responsibilities: projecting a professional image at all times while maintaining productivity, regulating the flow of patients through the office, and controlling the stress level of the office staff. Good dental office administrators are worth their weight in gold, not only to dentists but to their patients as well.

THE DENTAL OFFICE ENVIRONMENT

The dental office environment should be welcoming and comforting to the patient. Dental offices are no longer the cold and sterile places that they once were. Office design and colours are usually carefully planned and the psychological needs of the patient are considered. Many offices are decorated in soft, soothing colours and the clinical area is usually separated from the reception area. The terms "reception area" or "greeting area" replace the obsolete term "waiting room." The latter implies that patients should expect to wait for their appointments.

The reception area should be kept clean and tidy at all times. It is helpful if there is a play area where small children can occupy themselves. Many reception areas will contain an aquarium. This creates a distraction while promoting a peaceful and calm setting. It is important to direct the patient's attention away from a potentially stressful situation to a less threatening one. Waiting to see the dentist can provoke anxiety and fear in the patient, resulting in a less successful visit. Diversion, or turning attention away from a stress producing stimulus, is commonly used in dental offices. Treatment is generally more successful and recovery time is enhanced when the patient is relaxed and cooperative.

Music should be kept at a comfortable level, and soft, easy-listening music is recommended. Many dentists prefer classical music for its soothing effect.

If the reception area is untidy, the administrator should take the time to tidy up. This is a good opportunity to make sure that the magazines are not outdated. Many offices have magazines that are from years gone by. These create the impression that the dental treatment received there will also be outdated.

It is important for the dental office administrator to assume ownership of the job. To be an effective team member, you must remember one thing: there is no such thing as "It is not my job!" You must imagine that you are welcoming friends into your own living room. If you truly feel a sense of ownership for your position, you will willingly create a comfortable environment for guests.

PROTECTING THE PATIENTS

Most modern dental treatment rooms or operatories have "rear delivery systems" where the handpieces and instruments are behind the patient's head and not in full view. This helps to reduce the anxiety level of the patient. Patients are usually provided with sunglasses, not just for comfort from the glare of the bright light, but also for their protection during dental procedures when pieces of dental material can become airborne. A lead apron with an attached thyroid collar is used during dental x-ray procedures.

Patients should be assured that proper sterilization and infection control guidelines are followed. The clinical service providers must adhere to strict procedures to avoid contamination. These methods of risk management help to protect the patient, the clinical staff, and the administrative staff members.

The clinical and financial record of each patient must be kept strictly confidential at all times. Patients have a legal right to privacy, which cannot be violated by either the clinical or the administrative dental team.

PERSONAL QUALITIES

People who choose health care as a career are most often people who enjoy working with the public and are *helpers*. These qualities, along with many others, are what make them well suited for the position of a dental office administrator.

A positive attitude is absolutely essential. A good administrator feels good about him or herself, and demonstrates and promotes the value of good dental care. Body language speaks louder than words, and the simplest form of body language is a smile. A smile conveys warmth and gains the trust of the patient. It is the universal sign of acceptance. The patient needs to feel accepted, listened to, and understood.

It is important to remember that patients may be experiencing discomfort, anxiety, and lack of trust. These are barriers to communication that can be lessened by a pleasant facial expression, open gestures, eye contact, and a pleasant voice. The most remarkable thing about smiling is that it is not just the receiver of the communication that feels good, but also the sender.

A sense of humour is not always essential, but it certainly helps to maintain a positive attitude. Negative feelings are demonstrated in our body language in ways that are not always evident to us. Although it is important to behave responsibly, taking ourselves and others too seriously can rob us of the joy of communicating with others. Laughter is the best medicine and more health care professionals are realizing its beneficial effects on healing. Recovery is faster and home care instructions are usually followed when a patient has a positive attitude, and such an attitude can be modelled by health care providers.

Good physical health promotes emotional well-being. The dental office administrator should look and feel well. It does not create a positive impression on the patient if the dental office administrator looks sick, or if his or her personal dental health is not aesthetically pleasing. This demonstrates to the patient that the administrator does not value dental care; consequently, the patient will not be receptive to receiving dental care at that office.

The most rewarding aspects of our lives can be the most challenging. The dental office environment will be busy and sometimes stressful. The ability to deal with difficult people in a professional manner makes the dental office administrator a valuable asset to the practice. Personal problems should remain outside of the office environment. A team member who is constantly complaining creates a negative effect on the entire office.

Focusing on job responsibilities can help to put personal problems temporarily on hold. Often this will allow the bearer of such problems to look at them with a different perspective. Patients are the primary concern of the dental office administrator, as they keep the practice viable.

Enthusiasm is contagious and it helps to keep the staff working together toward a common goal, thereby creating a very positive over-all effect in the office. The objective is to make patients feel at ease, encourage referrals to the office, and create a positive experience for each of them. Good manners are essential also. Most of all, the dental administrator should remember to enjoy this challenging and rewarding career.

EMPLOYMENT OPPORTUNITIES

Many dental office administrators begin their careers by working in dental offices as receptionists. However, there are a variety of working environments available to highly skilled and motivated people. Some potential employers are the following:

- a dental practice
- an insurance company, as a claims adjudicator
- a dental supply company, as a customer service representative
- a computer software company
- a university or community college
- a research institution

The dental office administrator can explore these and many more diversified employment options. The key to success is having the required skills and educational background, maintaining personal integrity, and, above all, having a sincere desire to succeed.

ASSIGNMENT

Prepare an essay of four to six well-written paragraphs describing either a positive or a negative experience as a patient at a dental office. Use the points listed below as guidelines for preparation. If your dental experiences have been uneventful, solicit the help of friends or classmates. Most people are very willing to share their experiences, particularly if they were negative. Submit this assignment to your instructor for evaluation.

Consider the following:

- Briefly describe the event.
- How did you feel as a patient?
- What were your expectations as a patient?
- Describe whether or not your expectations were met.

If the event you are describing is negative, how could it be changed to a positive experience? If it is a positive experience, what do you feel made it so?

CHAPTER TWO

PATIENT COMMUNICATIONS

OBJECTIVE

At the end of this chapter, the student will be able to identify and describe the following: motivations for patients and staff, types of human behaviour, and common barriers to communication.

TOPICS

- applied psychology
- types of human behaviour
- Maslow's hierarchy of motivational needs
- what motivates patients
- understanding patient behaviour
- patient communications
- barriers to patient communications
- patient education regarding office policy and financial arrangements

---

APPLIED PSYCHOLOGY

In order to learn the art of effective communication skills, it is essential to understand some basics of human behaviour through applied psychology. People who have chosen a career in dentistry should develop a thorough understanding of what motivates patient behaviour. Applied psychology is the study of mental processes, feelings, and desires. It offers a method of predicting the reactions of people to the experiences of everyday life.

In order to understand patient behaviour, it is necessary to understand what motivates people. Motivation is an internal state or condition that activates behaviour and gives it direction. There are many theories about the factors that motivate human behaviour. Most psychologists agree that human behaviour is driven by psychological motives determined by an individual's needs. These needs can be related to survival or to the individual's happiness and state of well-being.

One popular theory of human motivational behaviour is described by Dr. Abraham Maslow. Maslow's theory suggests that our motives are organized in a hierarchy of needs arranged from the most basic to the most complex. This theory states that if the lower needs are not met, the higher needs remain dormant. As each level of needs is met, higher level motives become active and affect behaviour.

Maslow's hierarchy of motivational needs is usually shown as a pyramid; the lowest and most basic needs are at the bottom of the structure and the highest needs are at the top.

EXHIBIT 2.1 **MASLOW'S HIERARCHY OF BASIC MOTIVATIONAL NEEDS**

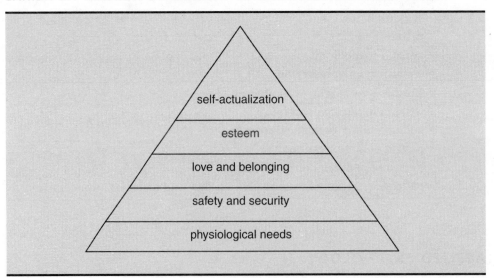

1. *Physiological needs.* The first and most basic human needs are for sleep, food, water, oxygen, and other requirements for life. These are our survival needs and, according to Maslow, only when these needs have been met will an individual be motivated by the next level or higher need.

2. *Safety and security.* The next higher needs include structure, law, order, and limits. We need to be free of fear, physical pain and danger, anxiety, chaos, and unknown threats. In a work setting, these needs could be related to things that threaten job security, such as discrimination or injustice.
3. *Love and belongingness.* This is our need for love, affection, and a feeling of belonging. People seek friendship and love through interaction with colleagues and friends. We strive for a place in the group.
4. *Esteem.* This is our need for a sense of self-worth, confidence, strength, capability, adequacy, and usefulness. Recognition and respect from our colleagues are important, because they relate to our ego or sense of self.
5. *Self-actualization.* This encompasses our need to develop to our fullest potentialities and capacities and our desire for self-fulfilment.

Although Maslow's theory is widely accepted, it represents a simplified model of human needs. Human beings are complex and we can be at different stages with different sets of needs at one time. It is very difficult to relate a particular behaviour to a single need at a given point. However, Maslow's theory does explain many facets of human motivation and, therefore, provides a perspective on how motivational factors affect human behaviour.

Our individual level in the hierarchy of motivational needs affects every aspect of our lives. For the patient, it affects awareness of the need for care and treatment. For the staff, it affects the ability to respond empathetically to patients and help them deal effectively with the stress of treatment.

Understanding Patient Behaviour

Factors which affect an individual's behaviour are derived from any one or a combination of the following factors.

Factors that affect behaviour:

- socioeconomic conditions
- culture
- current life situations
- previous dental or medical experiences
- attitudes and beliefs about personal health

Human values are developed before the age of 10. What is of value to one person may not be to another. For example, one person may clearly see the value of proper nutrition, exercise, or dental care, whereas another may not care about these things. Values are closely related to a person's *felt* needs, and they are intrinsic motivators.

A felt need is one the patient feels at the moment, a priority. This is a real need of the patient that affects his or her attitude toward dental health care. Felt needs are temporary, in the sense that when they are satisfied, they no longer exist; however, a value is developed early in life and maintained as a lifelong characteristic.

For example, a patient may complain bitterly about spending $80 on a preventive recall appointment and cleaning twice a year. The same patient could be spending more to improve personal appearance and self-esteem at a health club. Is the patient motivated because of the benefits of physical well-being only (a need to feel good), or to maintain an aesthetically pleasing body (a personal value)? Perhaps a combination of reasons is involved.

It is the responsibility of the dental team to help patients realize that the mouth is one of the most important parts of our digestive system. Therefore, proper dental fitness provides an individual with good health and a feeling of well-being and is aesthetically pleasing. A smile is one of the first features that is noticed by others, and having a healthy smile can enhance one's self-esteem. In order to develop a treatment program that the patient is comfortable with, it is important to discover what the patient values. The patient should feel that he or she is being listened to and understood.

A dental office environment is usually one of high fear and low trust. For many patients, the prospect of a visit to the dentist can create fear. Fear of pain is a learned response.

In the 1890s, Russian physiologist Ivan Pavlov, conducting research on the digestion of dogs, discovered the theory of "conditioned response" as an incidental finding.

Essentially, he believed that conditioning provoked a response and motivated behaviour. Pavlov conditioned the dogs to salivate at the sound of a bell through repeated exposure to the stimulus (the bell) at each feeding time. Conditioning can cause a predictable response in human behaviour through repeated exposure to a stimulus.

For dental patients, fear is a response to the expectation of discomfort. This fear response places the patient in a stress state. The emotional elements of this state can cause extreme sensitivity in the body, and as a result, the patient becomes defensive and uncooperative. This makes treatment difficult.

Responses will vary according to the personality and background of the patient. The patient's anxieties may result in hostile, irrational, and inappropriate behaviour. Because aggressive behaviour can be merely an expression of the patient's anxieties, it should not be taken personally by the dental office staff.

The fear of a dental visit can be the result of pain from past experience or fear of the unknown. Understanding the patient's cultural and socioeconomic background and current life situations, including any stresses, conflicts, and anxieties, will be helpful in coping with patient behaviour. It may be helpful to know something about previous dental treatments, as well as the reason for the current visit.

Negative psychological reactions are characterized by the patient being tense, suspicious, apprehensive, and resistant to suggested treatment. It is important to encourage trust and allay fear, remembering that trust is voluntary vulnerability.

Human behaviour can be categorized as psychotic, neurotic, or normal. These terms describe the approximate level of social adjustment an individual has achieved. Psychotic behaviour is usually severe, intense, and violently antisocial. Psychotic patients are usually hospitalized for their own protection.

A patient with neurotic behaviour is considered "maladjusted," or able to make a moderate social adjustment. As a society, we will accept neurotic behaviour within certain limits.

The following are examples of neurotic behaviour:

1. Depression—characterized by exaggerated sadness, reduced activity, fatigue with no physical cause.
2. Hysteria—characterized by excessive emotional reactions and by some physical conditions such as fainting.
3. Hypochondria—characterized by an unusual concern for one's physical health.
4. Phobia—characterized by an inordinate fear of specific situations.

In normal behaviour, a person is able to make a social adjustment that is better than moderate. The average normal patient is likely to be cooperative, relaxed, and friendly, will react to discomfort without showing fear or anxiety, and will fulfil home care and postoperative instructions.

Defence Mechanisms

Patients will react to a stressful situation with defence mechanisms. These are healthy and useful reactions unless carried to the extreme. A defence mechanism helps one cope with the stress of receiving treatment.

1. *Repression.* People temporarily forget things that produce tension or pain.
2. *Rationalization.* Some people make plausible excuses for irresponsible behaviour (e.g., missing appointments).
3. *Procrastination.* Avoiding an upsetting situation postpones the problem for as long as possible.
4. *Diversion.* Turning attention away from the unpleasant stimulus to one which does not produce tension (e.g., earphones, soft music, TV, a fish tank) is a very useful psychological defence mechanism for dental offices.
5. *Affiliation.* When people feel threatened, they prefer not to be alone and would rather be with friends than strangers. This is a normal coping mechanism. As a matter of courtesy, when a patient arrives, you should greet him or her promptly and pleasantly by name. It is reassuring to be called by one's own name and provides a feeling of worth and affiliation.
6. *Control.* People differ in degrees to which they try to control threatening situations. Some people prefer to control, and some to be controlled. A very important way in which patients can retain control is through communication during treatment.
7. *Rehearsal.* One can mentally go through a situation before it actually occurs. For example, athletes are renowned for their rehearsal techniques, also known as mental programming. Rehearsal is particularly important for children in the dental practice, as long as it is based on information and not imagination.

COMMUNICATION SKILLS

Just as important as understanding patient behaviour is the art of communication with people. Not only should you develop a positive attitude toward attending to the needs of others, but also you must consider the attitude of the patient being cared for. Why is it so important to determine the patient's values and outlook? When the attitude of the patient is considered, there is a greater opportunity for the patient to take responsibility for his or her own health. There is more willingness to accept the treatment recommended and participate in the recovery. Therefore, recovery and healing are more successful. The objective is to develop a relationship in which the patient is an active participant. Such relationships can be developed when the dental team meets the patient without judgment. It is important to avoid barriers to communication before they are built.

To be successful at interpersonal relationships, the dental team members should be in good physical and mental health and have enough self-esteem to give readily to others. Developing and maintaining effective communication skills are essential functions of the dental team, as approximately 90 percent of the working day is spent communicating with others.

Qualities of Good Communicators

1. Good physical and mental health.
2. A sense of confidence, understanding your job and doing it with pride.
3. A well-developed sense of personal identity.
4. A positive attitude toward yourself and others.
5. Empathy, the ability to understand the feelings of others.
6. The ability to interpret communications and to judge consequences.
7. The maturity to accept responsibility for your own conduct and efforts.

A simplified model of communication consists of a sender, a channel (method of communication), and a receiver. Communications are meaningless if the transfer from sender to receiver breaks down. We communicate by means of words, facial expression, appearance, voice inflection, and body language. The messages that we communicate through our body language can have broad implications. For example, lack of eye contact can send a message undermining the trust and credibility of the sender. If the source of the communication is considered to be credible, the influence on behaviour will be greater.

Encoding the communication is the process of putting the message into a form that the receiver will understand. For communications to be effective, they should be brief, focused, and timed appropriately.

Equally important is the channel of communication selected—for example, a written note, telephone call, or face-to-face conversation.

Appropriate channelling can help to enhance the acceptance and understanding of the message. Ineffective channelling can result in lack of attention to the message, regardless of the credibility of the sender.

The receiver of the communication is responsible for decoding the message and attaching meaning to it. It is crucial that the sender and the receiver of the communication are speaking the same language. For instance, you should not try to impress a patient with your technical knowledge using complicated dental terminology that the patient does not understand. This will create a barrier to communication and is simply poor manners.

The receiver of the information is subject to many influences, as is the sender. Both the sender and receiver of the communication are responsible for the accurate processing of information. In oral communications, paraphrasing provides instant feedback for the sender. It lets the sender know that he or she is being understood and that the communication is being coded or expressed appropriately. It allows the sender the opportunity to make adjustments.

Oral communications are those received by the ear; however, it is estimated that 90 percent of spoken words are not heard. Unspoken aspects of communication are perceived at a subconscious level. The total impact of a message depends on the voice tone of the sender, facial expression, and body language.

The body gestures of the dental office administrator should be open, caring, and communicative. Patients have a right to be greeted with a smile and feel that they are being welcomed to the practice. Acceptance of the proposed treatment is directly related to how the information was communicated. Therefore, excellent communication skills can enhance the financial productivity of a practice, whereas poor communication skills can create a negative impression on patients and result in nonacceptance of proposed treatment.

The entire dental team should be sensitive to their own body language, that is, the messages conveyed through movements and gestures. It is equally important to be sensitive to clues that are conveyed through the patient's body language. For example, crossed arms subconsciously indicate that the communication process is closed.

Listening is one of the most difficult acts in communication. It requires concentration and commitment. It requires that you tune the world out and tune the patient in.

Responsive listening is being sensitive to the feelings and needs that the patient is expressing. An effective, responsive listener will let the patient take the conversational lead and be sensitive to signals indicating that the patient wants to change topics or terminate the conversation. With practice, the dental team members can learn to recognize signals and practice high quality communication skills.

Effective communications will assist the dental office administrator to achieve and maintain control of administrative tasks through education of the dental patient. You will be more successful in obtaining a thorough medical history once a basis of trust has been established. Through proper encoding, channelling, and being sensitive to the body language of the patient, you can provide positive reinforcement and feedback regarding the dental treatment. Once trust has been established, you have the opportunity to educate the patient regarding office policies and procedures.

It is crucial for the dental office administrator to believe in the value of the service being performed by the dental professional. It would be beneficial for the office administrator to observe and understand what occurs during clinical procedures, since many patients will ask the administrator questions rather than the dentist. For example, patients may ask, "Why do I need this crown?" or "Why do I need periodontal surgery?" To help the patient understand the value of the treatment and to promote the dentistry that is being offered, the

TABLE 2.1 EXAMPLES OF POSITIVE COMMUNICATIONS

AVOID USING	CHANGE TO
Waiting room	Reception and/or greeting area
Dental work	Treatment
Filling	Restoration
File the tooth	Prepare the tooth
Price	Fee
Cost	Investment
The dentist would like . . .	The dentist recommends . . .
Checkup	Examination
Do you understand?	How do you feel about . . .?
Cancellation	Change in schedule
The dentist is running behind.	The dentist has had an interruption.
When would you like to come in?	Do you prefer a.m. or p.m.?

administrator should believe in the quality of care that is provided at that office. All dental team members should be consistent with their communications and familiar with the philosophy of the office.

Barriers to Patient Communications

Patients need to feel that they are active participants in their own wellness. One important barrier to communication can occur when they feel dehumanized, as if they are part of an assembly line. If members of the dental team know something unique about each patient and refer to him or her by name during verbal communications, the patient feels cared about as a person.

Dental team members will communicate with each other using dental terminology that is not always easily understood by the patient. This can sound intimidating and condescending. Complicated dental terminology does not belong in patient communications. Everyday terms should be used whenever possible, and explanation of all dental procedures should be offered before treatment is started.

Financial concerns can be quite distressing to a patient and create an unnecessary barrier to communication. It is important for the dental office administrator to experience empathy, to understand how the patient feels. Financial information is as personal and confidential as all medical information. Tact and understanding will help to reduce any barrier; however, the administrator must also be very definite about the payment policies of the practice. You should offer help to the patient regarding financial arrangements, dental insurance procedures, and so on, while maintaining a warm and professional attitude and allowing the patient to make an informed decision.

Fear of treatment is probably one of the most difficult barriers to overcome in patient communications. The administrator should ask the patient how long it has been since the last dental examination and what past experiences have been like. Thank the patient for sharing the experience and offer reassurance of providing the best possible care while minimizing discomfort. Explain to the patient how modern dental equipment and technologies have helped to improve a patient's dental experience. Offer further reassurance to the patient by discussing the sterilization procedures. This is sometimes an underlying concern.

Warmth and friendliness among staff members can reduce many barriers to communication. If there are tensions between staff members, patients pick up on them. A negative atmosphere in the office can cause the patient to feel uncomfortable and nervous. It is important to maintain a relaxed environment in which the dental team truly enjoys working.

Overcoming barriers to communication and practising excellent communication skills will be a major part of the job responsibilities of the dental office administrator. This process can be challenging and rewarding.

Practising Communication Skills With New Patients

When a new patient enters the practice, it is an opportunity to communicate the policies and procedures of the dental office. During the new patient interview, the office administrator can receive valuable information that may assist the dentist in identifying the needs of the patient and recommending the appropriate treatment. It is essential to listen to the patient to determine what is important to him or her.

It is a service to patients to ask how they feel about their smile or whether there is anything that they would like to change. Often, patients can simply be unaware that something can be done to change their smile. The dental office administrator should remember to ask questions and then listen to the answers without interrupting.

At the time of the new patient interview, the administrator should ask patients if they have dental insurance. This is an opportunity to educate them regarding the payment policy of the office and to offer assistance in understanding their dental insurance benefits and receiving reimbursement as efficiently as possible.

Patients should be made aware of the office hours and emergency number, and of the importance of keeping scheduled appointments and providing the office with adequate notice when a change in schedule is necessary. When the new patient interview is concluded, the dental office administrator should ask patients if they feel that everything has been explained. Patients need to know that they are being dealt with honestly and that they will receive quality service. They need to know that the dental team members care about their dental health and are available when needed. Patients do not care about how much you know until they know how much you care.

ASSIGNMENT

Think about your most recent dental appointment. Briefly describe the atmosphere of the office and the communications dynamics. What, if anything, would you have done differently?

Describe some of the positive communications that were encountered and some of the negative communications.

CHAPTER THREE

DENTAL TERMINOLOGY

OBJECTIVE

At the end of this chapter, the student will be able to identify and describe the following: prefixes, suffixes, root words, translation of dental terminology, spelling of dental terms, the components of terms, and rules for combining word parts to form dental terms.

TOPICS

- prefixes, suffixes, and root words
- pronouncing dental words
- building dental terms
- dental abbreviations
- practice exercises
- dental specialties
- glossary of dental terms

WORD FORMATION

It is important for a dental office administrator to learn the "language" of dentistry. Each area of dentistry will present terms that may be unfamiliar. This chapter provides a method of applying the principle of word building. This method involves building dental terms by recognizing the Greek and Latin word parts from which dental terms originate and joining these word parts by using combining forms. Most dental terms can be analyzed for their meaning by dividing them into their component parts and determining the meaning for each part.

As each new dental term is introduced, it is helpful to write it down on a separate piece of paper. This will reinforce the visual recognition of the word and the correct spelling. Pronouncing dental terms correctly will assist in spelling them correctly and provide auditory recognition of the term.

A medical dictionary and an English dictionary (such as Nelson's, Oxford's or Webster's) will be helpful. Consult the dictionary frequently for spelling and definitions.

Word Parts

All words have a word *root*. This is the foundation of a word, which gives the main idea or major meaning. Compound words are made up of more than one word root and are usually joined with a combining vowel. The most commonly used combining vowel is *o*, although *a, e, i, u* and *y* may be encountered occasionally. The combination of a word root plus a combining vowel is known as a combining form.

A **prefix** is a syllable or syllables placed before a word or word root to alter its meaning or create a new word. For example, if the prefix *re* is added to the word root *play*, a new word, *replay*, is created with a new meaning.

A **suffix** is a syllable or syllables placed at the end of a word root to alter its meaning and create a new word. For example, if the suffix *er* is added to the word root *play*, a new word, *player*, is created; it means one who plays.

Micr is the word root meaning small. *Micr/o* is the combining form. *Scope* is a suffix meaning instrument used to view. Thus, *microscope* is a term meaning instrument used to view small things.

When joining word roots using combining forms, if another word root begins with a vowel, sometimes the combining vowel is dropped. For example: *card/i* is the combining form meaning heart; *itis* is the suffix meaning inflammation. When these two word parts are joined the *i* in the combining form *card/i* is dropped to create the word *carditis* (not *cardi/itis*). Analyze the following terms:

1. carditis—inflammation of the heart
2. cephalitis—inflammation of the head
3. microcephalic—abnormally small head

Numbers

Uni and *mono* both mean one. A unicycle has one wheel. Monochrome means one colour.

Bi means two. A biscuspid is a tooth that has two cusps (or rounded surfaces).

Tri means three. A tricycle has three wheels.

Quad means four. Quadriplegia means paralysis of all four limbs.

Quint means five. Five babies born at the same time are known as quintuplets.

Sext means six. A sextuplet is one of six children born of a single gestation.

Sept means seven. This stems from the Latin word septum. A woman who has given birth to seven infants is known as a septipara.

Octa means eight. An octagon is a geometric shape which has eight sides.

Nona means ninth. Symptoms that appear every ninth day are called nonan.

Deca means ten. A decade is a period of ten years.

Cent means one hundred. One hundredth of a metre is a centimetre. An anthropod which is thought to have one hundred feet is called a centipede.

Milli means one thousand. A millimetre is one thousandth of a metre.

Kilo also means one thousand. Kilogram means one thousand grams.

Colours

Erythr/o is the combining form meaning red. An erythrocyte is a red blood cell.

Melan/o is the combining form meaning black. *Oma* is the suffix meaning tumour. Melanin is a black pigment that is contained in the skin. A melanoma is a cancerous tumour of the melanin—literally, black tumour.

Cyan/o is the combining form meaning blue. The suffix for condition is *osis*. A patient deprived of oxygen will exhibit a bluish tinge to the skin. This condition is called cyanosis. This is most evident when the lips turn blue.

Xanth/o is the combining form meaning yellow. *Dont* is the word part meaning tooth. A xanthodont is someone who has yellow teeth.

Leuk/o is the combining form for white. A leukocyte is a white blood cell.

Chlor/o is the combining form meaning green. Chloropia is a visual defect in which all things appear green.

GLOSSARY OF DENTAL TERMS

abutment	The anchorage tooth for a bridge. The supporting end of a bridge is the abutment.
acrylic restoration	Tooth repair using a synthetic plastic, acrylic, resin, or composite usually used to fill the anterior teeth. A white or coloured filling is usually an acrylic restoration.
alveolectomy	The surgical removal of part of the alveolar process. The suffix *ectomy* means to excise or surgically remove.
amalgam	The material replacing the lost part of the tooth or the diseased portion of the tooth. A mixture of silver and tin with mercury and some copper and zinc.
anterior teeth	Situated in front, referring to the upper and lower teeth located in the front area of the mouth. The upper and lower central incisors are examples of anterior teeth.
antrum lavage	Washing out of the sinus cavity by entering through the nose or mouth.
apex	The root end of any tooth.
apical curettage	The surgical cleaning and scraping of diseased tissue surrounding the end of the root. Apical refers to the apex. Curettage means to clean.
apicoectomy	Removal of the apex of a tooth root.
appliance	A device used to provide function or therapeutic effect to control oral habits. A night guard used to control grinding is a dental appliance.
articulator	A mechanical device which simulates the relationship and movement of the jaw. Articulate means to come together.

bacterial	Presence of living cells which cause disease. Plaque is a bacterial substance.
bicuspids	Two teeth next to the cuspids.
biopsy	Removal of a tissue specimen or other material from the living body for microscopic examination of it to aid in establishing a diagnosis.
bitewing	A cavity-detecting radiograph showing interproximal surfaces between the teeth. Two bitewing radiographs are usually taken at recall appointments.
bleaching	The use of a chemical oxidizing agent to lighten tooth discolourations.
bruxism	The unnatural grinding of teeth. Many dental problems are the result of bruxism.
buccal	Pertaining to or adjacent to the cheek. The outer surface of posterior teeth is the buccal surface.
calculus	Mineralized plaque on the surface of the teeth. Also called tartar. Proper cleansing of teeth can help to control calculus.
canal	The portion of the root that contains the pulp tissue and is surrounded by dentin.
caries	Dental decay. Dentists remove decay from teeth before placing a restoration.
cariogenic	A substance that will cause caries or dental decay. Sugar is a cariogenic substance.
carious	Carious is the adjectival form of caries. Before a restoration is placed a dentist will remove the carious lesion.
cast metal post and core	A custom cast metal form inserted and cemented in the canal or root of the tooth. Designed to support an artificial crown when there is insufficient tooth structure to support it.
cast space maintainer	A mechanical prosthetic device to prevent the drifting of teeth where premature loss of a tooth (or teeth) has occurred.
cementum	A specialized, calcified connective tissue that covers the anatomic root of a tooth.
cephalometric film	An extra-oral radiograph of the head to assist in the evaluation of the patient's facial growth and development. *Cephalo* is the combining form meaning head. Therefore, an x-ray that measures the head is a cephalometric x-ray.

complete dentures	A dental prosthesis that replaces all of the natural dentition in the same arch.
complete series radiographs	A series of periapical radiographs showing all individual areas of the mouth, including the teeth roots and gums, also known as a full mouth series (FMS). Part of the new patient procedure may include taking an FMS.
composite restorations	Tooth repair using improved synthetic resins which remain colour fast and are stronger than other synthetic materials. Restorations on anterior or posterior teeth are usually composite restorations.
consultation	An appointment in which the dentist discusses with the patient an intended treatment plan or necessary dental treatment for a particular problem. A patient or the dentist may request a consultation to discuss treatment.
crown	That portion of a human tooth covered by enamel. Also, an artificial restoration which becomes the entire surface of the tooth above the gum line and which fits over a prepared tooth; may be made of porcelain, acrylic resin, metal, or a combination of these materials.
cuspids	One of the four pointed teeth in humans, situated one on each side of each jaw. These are also known as the canines or "eye teeth."
deciduous teeth	Teeth that break through the gums and will be shed and replaced by permanent teeth. Also called primary teeth or baby teeth. Deciduous teeth begin to shed at approximately age 6.
dental arch	That part of the upper and lower jaw which contains soft and hard tissue supporting the natural teeth or a fabrication appliance.
dental pulp	Occupies a hollow space called the pulp chamber and root canal inside the centre of the tooth.
dentin	The portion of the tooth that lies subjacent to the enamel and cementum.
dentition	All of the teeth in the dental arches. A child under 6 years of age will have a deciduous dentition. An adolescent will have a mixed dentition, whereas an adult will have a permanent dentition.
diagnostic casts	A negative likeness of dental structures for the purpose of study and treatment planning. Can be constructed of plaster or stone.
distal	The tooth surface that is farthest away from the midline of the dental arch.

edentulous	Without teeth. A patient who has had all of their teeth removed is known as edentulous.
enamel	A hard, glistening white substance that covers the crown of the tooth. The hardest substance in the human body.
endodontics	That specialty in dentistry that treats disease of the pulp and of the periapical tissue which supports the end of the root of the tooth. The procedure codes for root canal therapy are found under the category of endodontics.
extra-oral film	A picture which examines all the external structures of the oral cavity. Placed outside the mouth.
fluoride	A treatment to reduce caries activity; may be by means of water supply; oral hygiene preparations for home use, or topical applications for the purpose of prophylaxis. Be careful of the spelling of this word.
fractures	A break in continuity of bone. In the oral region it is most frequently seen in teeth and related structures.
frenectomy	Excision of the fold of tissue which connects the cheeks and lips to the upper and lower dental arch and limits their movement. If the frenum is too short, the dentist will need to perform a frenectomy.
frenum	A fold of mucous membrane attaching the cheeks and lips to the upper and lower jaw. The phrase "tongue tied" can mean that the frenum is too short, resulting in restricted movement of the tongue.
gingiva	The fibrous tissue covered by mucous membrane that immediately surrounds the teeth, also called the gums.
gingivectomy	When the gum tissue becomes separated from the tooth wall it is sometimes necessary to surgically remove the diseased and infected portion, creating a new gum line. The suffix *ectomy* means surgical removal.
gingivitis	Any inflammation of the gingival tissue.
gingivoplasty	Surgical shaping of the gum tissue in order to support the teeth so that they can perform their normal function.
glossitis	Inflammation of the tongue. *Glosso* is the combining form meaning tongue.
gold foil restoration	A filling which is produced from pure gold rolled into thin sheets. It is condensed into the prepared surface piece by piece.

hemisection	Cutting through the crown of the tooth into the root area to remove the affected portion of the crown and root.
immediate dentures	Type of denture constructed for insertion immediately following removal of the natural anterior teeth.
incisors	A cutting tooth. One of the four anterior teeth of either jaw. Central incisors are the centre front teeth, and lateral incisors are on either side of the centrals.
inlay	A restoration of metal, fired porcelain, or plastic made to fit a tapered cavity preparation.
interproximal	Interproximal means between two proximal surfaces (i.e., the mesial and distal). A bitewing radiograph is helpful to examine the interproximal spaces between teeth.
intra-oral films	A radiograph which examines inside the oral cavity. Taken from inside the mouth.
intravenous	Intravenous means within the vein. The administration of drugs within the vein will be an intravenous injection.
labial	Pertaining to the lip. The tooth surface on anterior teeth that touches the lip is the labial surface.
lingual	Pertaining to the tongue. The tooth surface that touches the tongue is known as the lingual surface.
local anaesthesia	Loss of feeling or sensation in a localized area.
mandible	The lower jaw.
mandibular	The adjectival form for mandible. This refers to the teeth in the lower jaw.
mastication	Chewing.
mesial	Facing toward the midline of the body or toward the centre of the dental arch. The tooth surface that faces the midline is the mesial surface.
mixed dentition	A group of teeth that consist of a mixture of adult teeth and deciduous teeth; usually from the ages of 6 to 12 years.
molars	Large teeth at the back of the mouth, used to grind and crush food. The first permanent molars erupt at approximately age 6.
morphology	The branch of biology that deals with the form and structure of an organism or part. *Morph* is the root word meaning form; *ology* is a suffix meaning study of. The

	study of teeth and the supporting structures is known as dental morphology.
narcotic	A drug, usually with strong analgesic action and an addiction potential. A narcotic is a drug that can induce sleep.
necrosis	Death of a cell or group of cells.
necrotic	The adjectival form of necrosis. When tissue is considered to be dead it is called necrotic tissue.
nitrous oxide and oxygen	N_2O, conscious sedation, sometimes referred to as laughing gas, administered through an inhalant.
nutrition	Food intake and how the body utilizes it. Proper nutrition can affect dental health.
obturator	A prosthesis used to close an opening in the palate.
occlusal	The act of closing teeth on opposing arches together; chewing surface of posterior teeth. The chewing surface of a posterior tooth is the occlusal surface.
occlusal equilibration	Modification of occlusal surfaces with intent to balance the bite.
occlusal film	Radiograph used to show large areas of the bone of the skull that supports the upper and lower jaw.
onlay	A restoration that extends over one or more cusps and adjoining occlusal surfaces of the tooth.
oral hygiene instruction/oral self-care	Teaching patients the proper way to clean their teeth in order to eliminate decay and gum disease. Effective toothbrushing and flossing techniques. Oral hygiene instruction is part of every recall appointment.
oral pathology	The branch of medicine which deals with the causes and symptoms of oral disease. *Pathos* is the root word meaning disease and *ology* is the suffix meaning study of. The study of disease within the mouth is known as oral pathology.
organism	Any living body.
orthodontic	The speciality of dentistry which corrects abnormal arrangement of teeth and/or jaws, straightens them, and keeps them in correct position. Braces are a form of orthodontic treatment.
overbite	Vertical overlapping of upper teeth over lower ones.
overhang	Excess filling material projecting beyond cavity margins.

palate	Roof of the mouth. The roof of the mouth is further broken into the hard palate, which is the anterior portion, and the soft palate, which is in the back.
pallor	Paleness; absence of skin colouration.
panoramic film	A single radiographic film that shows the entire character and arrangement of the teeth and the surrounding gum and bone structure. Also called panorex or panalypse.
partial denture	A dental prosthesis constructed to fit over the gums and hold artificial teeth.
periapical radiograph	A dental x-ray that shows the roots or apex of the teeth and surrounding bone. *Peri* is a prefix meaning around *apical* is the adjectival form for apex.
periodontal disease	Disease which affects the supporting tissue of the teeth, such as the gums and bone surrounding the teeth. Patients who do not floss their teeth may be at risk for peridontal disease.
permanent dentition	The 32 teeth of adulthood that replace the primary teeth.
pharmacology	The science of drugs, including their use in therapeutics. A dental office administrator should have some understanding of pharmacology.
physiology	The study of tissue and organism behaviour.
pit and fissure sealants	Clear plastic material used to coat and seal the pits and fissures or the biting surfaces of the back teeth to protect them from decay. A preventive procedure that helps children through their cavity prone years.
plaque	A sticky, bacterial substance that accumulates on the teeth. Plaque is often responsible for caries and gingival inflammation.
pontic	The structure that replaces the missing tooth of a bridge and is attached to the abutment. Replaces the missing natural tooth. Pontic means false.
posterior teeth	Refers to the teeth at the back of the mouth, such as bicuspids and molars.
premolar	Bicuspid. When deciduous molars are shed in the deciduous dentition, bicuspids will replace them in the dental arch. Many dentists will refer to the bicuspid as the premolar.

primary	The first dentition (or deciduous dentition) consists of the primary teeth.
prophylaxis	A series of procedures whereby calculus, stain, and other accretions are removed from the teeth and the teeth are polished. Prophylaxis means prevention of disease. A six-month recall appointment will consist of scaling plus prophylaxis.
pulp	The substance made up of blood vessels and nerves that occupies the central portion of teeth. An endodontic procedure will include removal of all or part of the pulp.
pulpectomy	Surgical removal of the entire dental pulp.
pulpotomy	Pulp amputation. The suffix *otomy* means to cut into, incise. If the dentist removes part of the pulp the procedure is called pulpotomy.
radiograph	An image or picture produced on a film. *Radio* is a prefix which refers to radiation. The suffix *graph* means picture. Also known as x-ray.
radiology	That branch of medicine dealing with the diagnostic and therapeutic applications of radiation.
reline	To resurface the tissue side of a denture.
retentive pins	When most of a tooth is lost it is usually necessary to support the large filling with stainless steel pins—retentive pins—which are cemented or threaded into certain positions in the base of the tooth. Can also be used when the corner of a tooth has broken off to support a filling in that area.
root canal therapy	Treatment to remove the nerve of a tooth. Procedure done in endodontics.
scaling	The removal of calculus deposits from teeth.
sedation	The production of a sedative effect; the act or process of calming.
silicate restoration	Tooth repair using a hard, tooth-coloured material for restoring the anterior teeth.
socket	The bony cavity in the upper or lower arch of the jaw in which the root of a tooth is held.
splinting	Binding or joining of loose or weak teeth to one another to stabilize and strengthen them.
stainless steel crown	A preformed crown used to repair badly broken down teeth; usually in primary teeth.

sublingual	Pertaining to the region beneath the tongue. *Sub* is the prefix meaning below; *lingual* refers to the tongue. A medication that is administered below the tongue is a sublingual medication.
sulcus	A groove or depression that surrounds the teeth in the oral cavity. Proper tooth brushing will help to disturb the colonies of bacteria in the sulcus.
surgery	The branch of medicine which treats diseases, injuries, and deformities by operative methods.
syncope	Fainting. The "e" in this word is pronounced, i.e., sin-kop-ee. If a patient is about to faint they are experiencing syncope.
syndrome	A group of symptoms that occur together and characterize a disease. For example, Down's syndrome is the name used for a group of symptoms that are characteristic of trisomy 21.
tartar	The formation and collection on the surface of the teeth of mineralized plaque. Hardened plaque is tartar.
temporomandibular joint	Also called the TMJ. Area surrounding the joint which manipulates the opening and closing of the lower jaw and is situated at the end of the upper and lower arches near the ear. An improper bite and bruxism can affect this joint.
tissue	An aggregation of similarly specialized cells united in performance of a particular function.
torus	A bulging projection of bone.
toxic	Poisonous. A lethal dose of a drug is fatal, whereas a dosage that is not lethal is poisonous or toxic.
tranquillizer	Drugs designed to produce a calm and relaxed state without interfering with physical responsiveness or mental clarity. A patient may require a tranquillizer before treatment can commence.
vestibule	The cavity at the entrance to the oral cavity that lies between the teeth, lips, and cheek.
vestibular	The adjectival form of vestibule, referring to the tooth surface that faces the cheek or lips. This can also be known as the facial surface. Dental insurance companies prefer to use vestibular to describe a buccal or labial surface.
vitality test	Determines if the pulp of the tooth is dead or nonvital.

wound	An injury to the body caused by physical means.
x-ray	A radiograph; radiation characterized by wave lengths.
zinc oxide and eugenol	Also called ZOE. Material used for impressions, root canal, surgical dressings, temporary fillings, and cementing media.

ASSIGNMENT

Fill in the blanks:

1. Word parts are joined by a combining vowel which is usually an ___, but can be another vowel.

2. The word part that is placed at the beginning of a word to alter its meaning is a _____.

3. The word part that is placed at the end of a word to alter its meaning is a _____.

4. a. *Electr/o* is the combining form meaning electricity. *Cardi/o* is the combining form meaning heart. *Gram* is a suffix meaning record. Build a word meaning a record of the electrical activity of the heart. _____.

   b. *Graph* is the word part meaning instrument used to record. Build a term meaning instrument used to record the electrical activity of the heart. _____.

   c. *Graphy* is the word part meaning procedure or process of recording. Build a term meaning the process of recording the electrical activity of the heart. _____.

5. *Radi/o* is the combining form meaning radiant energy which is used for x-rays. The process of recording radiant energy is

   _____.

6. The film on which an image is produced through exposure to x-ray radiation is the material used to record dental x-rays. A dental x-ray is also known as a _____.

7. *Cephal/o* is the combining form meaning head. *Metric* is a suffix meaning pertaining to measurement. A dental x-ray that is used to measure the head, in particular, the relationship of the jaw, is known as a _____ x-ray.

8. *Stomat/o* is the combining form meaning mouth. *Itis* is the suffix meaning inflammation. Inflammation of the mouth is

    _____.

9. a. Cleaning the apical area of the tooth is _____.

    b. A tooth that has two cusps (or rounded surfaces) is a

    _____

    c. The anchorage tooth for a bridge is the _____.

    d. Silver coloured fillings that are used on posterior teeth are called

    _____.

    e. The root end of any tooth is its _____.

    f. The dental x-ray that reveals interproximal decay is known as a

    _____.

CHAPTER FOUR

TOOTH MORPHOLOGY

OBJECTIVE

At the end of this chapter, the student will be able to identify and describe the following: terms related to the oral structures, parts of the tooth structure and surrounding tissues, bone and soft tissue structures of the head and neck, surfaces of an anterior tooth and a posterior tooth, and the eruption cycle from the primary to the permanent dentition.

TOPICS

- oral structures and facial anatomy
- types of teeth
- structure of a tooth
- functions of anterior and posterior teeth
- tooth surfaces
- types of dentition: primary, mixed, permanent
- eruption cycle of teeth from deciduous to permanent

PARTS OF THE MOUTH

The mouth is one of the most important components of the digestive system. It prepares food for digestion by breaking it into smaller portions and mixing it with saliva. The lips protect the anterior opening of the mouth. The dental word root for lips is *labia*. The cheeks form the lateral walls of the mouth. The dental term for cheek is *buccal*. The palate is the horizontal structure which separates the mouth and the nasal cavity. The hard palate forms the anterior portion of the roof of the mouth and is also known as the bony palate. The soft palate forms the posterior portion of the roof. The uvula is a finger-like projection of the soft palate which extends downward from its posterior edge. The uvula is also known as the pendulous palate.

The space between the lips and cheeks externally and the teeth and gums internally is the vestibule. The facial surfaces of anterior and posterior teeth are known as the vestibular surfaces.

The muscular tongue occupies the floor of the mouth. The tongue has several bony attachments; two of these are to the hyoid bone and the styloid processes of the skull. The frenum is a fold of mucous membrane that connects two parts and serves to check the movement of the parts. The lingual frenum secures the tongue to the floor of the mouth and limits its posterior movements. The frenum of the lips attaches the lips to the alveolar mucosa and is located between the upper and lower central incisors.

Children are often born with an extremely short frenum. Speech is distorted when movement of the tongue is restricted. This congenital

EXHIBIT 4.1 PARTS OF THE MOUTH

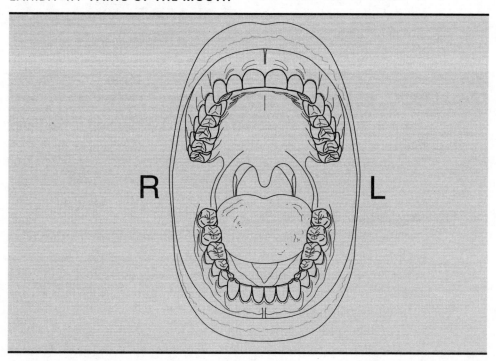

The DMD (Dental Management Document) and the DMD Emergency Treatment System have been reproduced with the permission of Dental Risk Management Systems Inc., which holds the copyright.

condition can be corrected surgically by cutting or excising the frenum. This surgical procedure is called a frenectomy. The indentation that extends from the nostrils to the vermilion border of the lips is called the philtrum.

As food enters the mouth, it is mixed with saliva and chewed. The process of chewing is called mastication. The cheeks and closed lips hold the food between the teeth during chewing. The tongue continually mixes food with saliva during chewing and initiates swallowing.

The teeth are rooted in sockets of the alveolar process, which is made up of the bony ridges that project from the jaw bone to anchor the teeth. The gums, or gingiva, cover the alveolar process and extend into each socket.

The upper jaw is the maxilla and the lower jaw is the mandible. The teeth are aligned into two dental arches, the maxillary arch and the mandibular arch. The U-shaped mandible is the strongest and largest bone of the face. The mandible is attached to the cranium by the ligaments of the temporomandibular joint (TMJ). This joint receives its name from two other bones that enter into its formation, the temporal bone and the mandible. The left and right temporomandibular joints function together. These joints are synovial joints that permit the specialized hinge and glide movements which provide different degrees of mouth opening.

Types of Teeth

There are four types of teeth, each of which performs different functions.

The **incisors** are designed for cutting. These teeth are located at the anterior portion of the mouth and consist of central incisors and lateral incisors. The incisors can cut through food without the application of much force.

The **cuspids** are also known as the **canines**. These teeth have a slightly thicker enamel and their function is for tearing. They have a larger crown than the incisors, but they usually come to a point. The roots of the cuspid are the longest in the dentition. The cuspids are the cornerstones of the dental arches.

The **bicuspids** are also sometimes referred to as the premolars because they are before the molars. They are called bicuspids because they have two cusps, which assist with grasping and tearing of food. They also have a broader chewing surface, which helps to grind food.

The **molars** are located in the posterior portion of the mouth and their purpose is to grind food. They are shorter and blunter than the other teeth, with a broader surface for chewing. A great deal of force is applied to the molars during mastication.

The function of each dental arch is directly related to the form and position of each tooth within that arch. Normal development and proper positioning determine the stability and efficiency of the oral cavity. If the teeth are not in proper position, the function and efficiency will be reduced. The misalignment of the jaw is called malocclusion. The term "occlude" means to come together, as in the chewing surfaces of opposing posterior teeth. Occlusion is the state of being closed. Malocclusion refers to teeth that are improperly positioned when the mouth is closed. Centric occlusion occurs when the jaws are closed in a position that produces maximum stable contact between the opposing surfaces of the maxillary and the mandibular teeth.

EXHIBIT 4.2 TYPES OF TEETH

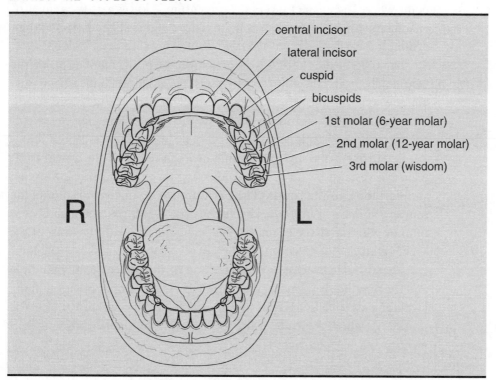

The DMD (Dental Management Document) and the DMD Emergency Treatment System have been reproduced with the permission of Dental Risk Management Systems Inc., which holds the copyright.

Structure of a Tooth

Each tooth (see Exhibit 4.3) consists of the enamel, cementum, dentin, pulp, and periodontal ligament and it is embedded in a bony socket called the alveolar process. The enamel is the hard bone-like substance that covers the crown of the tooth. Enamel is the hardest substance in the human body, comparable in hardness to quartz. Enamel protects the tooth against the wear and tear of chewing and against chemical substances that might dissolve the dentin. Enamel, unlike other body tissues, is unable to repair itself when damaged.

Dentin lies beneath the enamel and consists of dense connective tissue which extends over the entire tooth. It is less dense than enamel and yet more dense than bone. The internal surface of dentin forms the walls of the pulp cavity. In permanent teeth, dentin is pale yellow and somewhat transparent. Age-related attrition (the natural wearing of teeth) can cause dentin to be exposed, resulting in a yellowish appearance, particularly on the cutting edge of the lower incisors.

Cementum covers the root of the tooth, overlaying the dentin. The point where the enamel meets the cementum is known as the cemento-enamel junction. Cementum is light yellow and is slightly darker than dentin. It is easily distinguished from enamel because of its lack of lustre.

The pulp of the tooth is located within the pulp chamber inside the dentin. The pulp contains blood vessels, nerves, and connective tissue. Narrow extensions of the pulp pass through the root ends of the tooth. The root end of the tooth is known as the apex. These narrow extensions are the root canals.

Each root canal has an opening at its base called the apical foramen. Nerves and blood vessels connecting through the apical foramen supply blood to the tooth. The periodontal ligament surrounds the tooth to support it in its socket. It consists of soft tissue which is continuous with the tissue of the gingiva and connects with the bone of the socket wall.

The alveolar process is the extension of the bones of the mandible and the maxilla. It supports the teeth in their functional position in the jaws. The alveolar socket, or alveolus, is the cavity within the alveolar process in which the root of the tooth is held by the periodontal ligament.

The Eruption Cycle of Teeth

At approximately 6 months of age, the first teeth erupt into the dentition. These teeth are called deciduous. Eventually these teeth will be

EXHIBIT 4.3 **STRUCTURE OF A TOOTH**

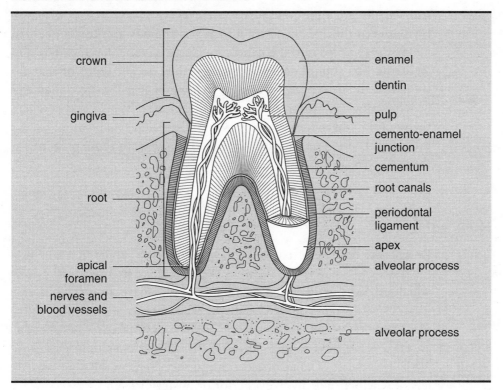

shed. The first dentition is called the primary dentition. The first primary teeth to erupt into the dentition are usually the upper and lower central incisors. New teeth will continue to erupt until there are a total of 20 teeth in the primary dentition. A full set should be present by approximately age 2.

At approximately 6 years of age, the primary teeth will become loose and the first permanent molars will erupt into the dentition. This is the beginning of the mixed dentition stage. This process of exfoliation, or shedding, occurs between 5 and 12 years of age. The next permanent molars to erupt into the dentition are the 12-year molars.

During the mixed dentition stage, children will have a combination of primary and permanent teeth. A child may experience problems with occlusion because of an irregular bite. As a result, some children may grind their teeth and may experience headaches. Problems with occlusion can sometimes be corrected with removable orthodontic appliances. However, orthodontic correction is usually not considered until the 12-year molars have erupted. The mixed dentition stage involves the cavity-prone years and good oral hygiene should be stressed along with preventive treatment.

Between the ages of 18 and 35 years, the wisdom teeth, or third molars, may erupt into the dentition. Not everyone develops wisdom teeth and one should not be alarmed if they do not erupt. If they do come into the dentition correctly, providing proper function, they will be left in the jaw. However, the human evolutionary process, in which the maxilla and mandible have become smaller, has resulted in less room for eruption of the wisdom teeth. If these teeth cause pressure on the jaw, extraction will be necessary.

Tooth Surfaces

Every tooth has five surfaces. Restoring a tooth to proper function may range from a small restoration on one surface to a larger restoration which involves many surfaces and actual reconstruction of the tooth itself. Dental professionals identify the type of restoration made by first identifying the tooth surfaces involved. Due to differences in function, anterior teeth have slightly different tooth surfaces than posterior teeth. The names of some of the tooth surfaces remain the same regardless of whether they involve anterior or posterior teeth.

Lingual The inside surface of every tooth that touches the tongue is known as the lingual surface. The lingual surface is the same on anterior and posterior teeth.

Mesial The mesial surface is the surface of a tooth that is facing toward, or closest to, the midline. The mesial surface is the same on anterior and posterior teeth.

Distal The distal surface is the surface of a tooth that is facing away from, or farthest away from, the midline. The distal surface is the posterior surface on either anterior or posterior teeth.

Proximal Proximal surfaces are surfaces that are directly adjacent to each other in the same arch. The mesial and distal surfaces are proximal surfaces. The space between the mesial surface of one tooth and the distal surface of an adjacent tooth is called the interproximal space.

Buccal The buccal surface is the surface which is immediately adjacent to the cheek on posterior teeth only. This is sometimes referred to as the facial surface.

Labial The labial surface is the surface positioned adjacent to the lip on anterior teeth only. This also may be referred to as the facial surface.

Vestibular Vestibular is a collective term which refers to the facial surface of an anterior or posterior tooth. Therefore, vestibular identifies either a labial or a buccal surface.

Occlusal The occlusal surface is the top surface, or chewing surface, of a posterior tooth. This surface has a broad base and is functional in chewing.

Incisal The incisal surface is the cutting surface, or edge, of anterior teeth. It is functional in cutting and tearing of food.

Each tooth surface is identified by the first letter of the name of the surface. For example: MODBL identifies the surfaces: mesial, occlusal, distal, buccal, and lingual. The suffix *al* of each word identifies that this is the adjectival form and describes the relationship of the surface to the dental arch. When joining more than one tooth surface in written communication, drop the suffix *al* and join the terms with the combining vowel *o*. For example: mesio-occlusodistobuccolingual. In order to distinguish the difference between a lingual (the surface touching the tongue) and a labial (the anterior surface that touches the lip) surface, add the next letter. La = labial, Li = lingual.

It is essential to know the anatomical names of each tooth surface to facilitate correct administration of dental insurance forms, correspondence, and communication within the dental community. A tooth surface noted incorrectly on an insurance form can result in the refusal of a dental claim, which causes inconvenience to the patient and might have legal implications for the dental practice.

ASSIGNMENT

1. How many teeth are in the permanent dentition?
2. What is the medical term which refers to the upper arch?
3. What is the medical term which refers to the lower arch?
4. How many teeth are in the primary dentition?
5. What is the chewing surface of a posterior tooth called?
6. What is the tooth surface that is toward the midline called?
7. What is the tooth surface that is furthest away from the midline called?
8. List and identify the surfaces of a posterior tooth and an anterior tooth.
9. Label the following diagram.

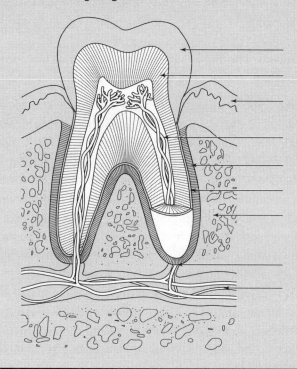

CHAPTER FIVE

TOOTH IDENTIFICATION AND NUMBERING SYSTEMS

OBJECTIVE

At the end of this chapter, the student will be able to identify and describe the following: the three systems of tooth identification and all teeth in the primary, mixed, and permanent dentition according to each tooth numbering system.

TOPICS

- Tooth identification systems
- International Tooth Numbering System
- Universal Tooth Numbering System
- Palmer's Identification System

IMPORTANCE OF TOOTH IDENTIFICATION

Methods of recording information on the clinical chart may vary from office to office, but it is necessary to understand and follow a consistent system of tooth identification. Dental charts are permanent legal documents and accuracy is essential. A forensic pathologist, for example, may need to rely on dental records to identify a victim or missing person. A system of instant identification should be practical and easily understood by all dental professionals.

Identification systems enhance the efficiency of dental claims adjudication. An adjudicator can instantly identify where the tooth is located in the mouth, whether it is a primary or permanent tooth, and the type of restoration involved. This information is recorded by the insurance company to prevent the duplication of claim payment. There are a variety of methods of identification available to the dental professional, and the three most commonly used systems are discussed in this chapter.

INTERNATIONAL TOOTH NUMBERING SYSTEM

The foremost identification system used throughout Canada is the International Tooth Numbering System. This system is the most efficient and easy to use. It is often called the two-digit numbering system. The first digit indicates the quadrant in which the tooth is located, and the second digit indicates where the tooth is located within the quadrant. The first digit also indicates whether the tooth is permanent or primary.

To understand the mechanics of this system, it is necessary to divide the mouth into four quadrants. When looking at dental charts, it helps to visualize the patient in the dental chair with his or her mouth open. Imagine that there is a line through the centre of the skull cutting it into right and left halves. This imaginary line is known as the midsagittal plane or the midline.

EXHIBIT 5.1 MIDLINE

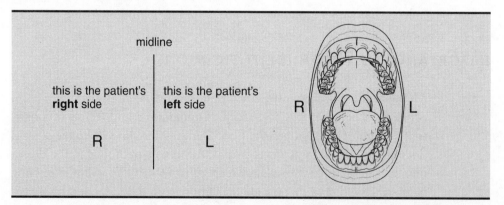

The DMD (Dental Management Document) and the DMD Emergency Treatment System have been reproduced with the permission of Dental Risk Management Systems Inc., which holds the copyright.

The second imaginary line or plane runs along the occlusal surfaces of the teeth, separating the jaw into upper and lower halves. This is known as the transverse plane.

The mouth is now divided into four quadrants. An adult dentition consists of 32 teeth; therefore, each quadrant will contain eight teeth.

Beginning at the midline of the upper right quadrant, the teeth are as follows:

- central incisor
- lateral incisor
- cuspid

EXHIBIT 5.2 **TRANSVERSE PLANE**

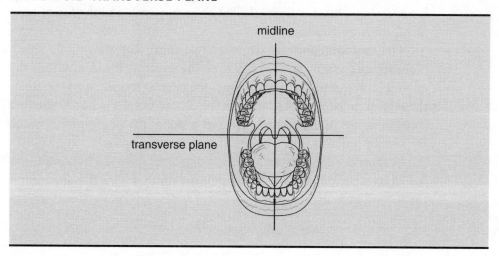

EXHIBIT 5.3 **QUADRANTS**

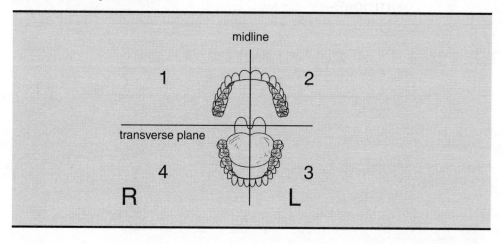

- first bicuspid (premolar)
- second bicuspid (premolar)
- first molar (6-year molar)
- second molar (12-year molar)
- third molar or wisdom tooth

Dentists will begin an examination in the upper right quadrant and continue in a clockwise direction. Each numbering system follows this basic technique.

The first number of the International Tooth Numbering System identifies the quadrant where the tooth is located. Beginning in the upper right quadrant, this is identified as quadrant 1. Proceeding in a clockwise direction, the upper left quadrant is identified as 2. The lower left quadrant is then labelled as quadrant 3, and the lower right quadrant is quadrant 4.

The second number in the two-digit International Tooth Numbering System identifies where the tooth is located within the quadrant. Beginning at the midline, the central incisor is tooth no. 1, the lateral incisor would be tooth no. 2, the cuspid is no. 3, the first bicuspid is no. 4, the second bicuspid is no. 5, the first molar is no. 6, the second molar is no. 7, and the third molar is no. 8.

In this two-digit system, the first digit identifies the quadrant, followed by a period, and the number of the tooth within the quadrant is the second number.

EXHIBIT 5.4 INTERNATIONAL TOOTH NUMBERING SYSTEM: ADULT DENTITION

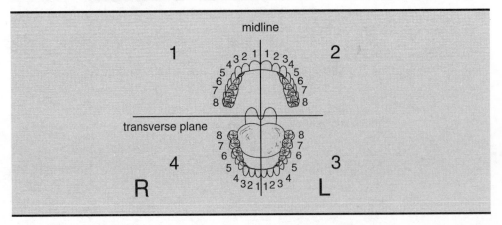

For example, the upper right central incisor would be identified as tooth no.1.1 according to this tooth numbering system. The upper left first bicuspid is tooth no. 2.4. The lower left lateral incisor would be tooth no. 3.2, and the lower right first molar would be tooth no. 4.6.

It is important when using this tooth numbering system orally to identify each number. For example you should say (tooth number) "one one," "two four," "three two," or "four six," rather than (tooth number) "eleven," "twenty-four," "thirty-two," or "forty-six."

The International Tooth Numbering System also provides a means to distinguish between a permanent and a primary tooth. The primary dentition contains only 20 teeth; therefore, there are five teeth in each quadrant. The basic format is the same in that each quadrant is identified by number beginning in the upper right quadrant and numbering in a clockwise direction. The main difference, however, is that the upper right quadrant is now quadrant 5. The upper left quadrant is quadrant 6, the lower left quadrant is quadrant 7, and the lower right quadrant is quadrant 8.

Beginning at the midline, the central incisor is tooth no. 1. The lateral incisor is tooth no. 2, the cuspid is tooth no. 3, and the primary molars are no. 4 and no. 5.

For example, the upper right primary central incisor is tooth no. 5.1. The upper left primary lateral incisor is tooth no. 6.2. The lower left primary cuspid is tooth no. 7.3. The lower right primary first molar is tooth no. 8.4.

EXHIBIT 5.5 **INTERNATIONAL TOOTH NUMBERING SYSTEM: PRIMARY DENTITION**

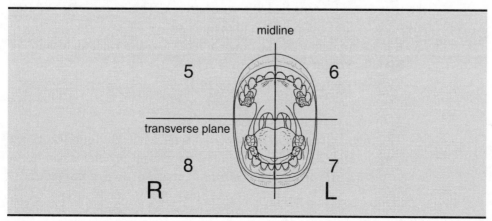

It is not necessary to memorize which teeth belong in which quadrant and their respective tooth numbers. The process of learning this system is similar to that of learning how to read a map.

UNIVERSAL TOOTH NUMBERING SYSTEM

The Universal Tooth Numbering System is a method of numbering teeth that is widely accepted in the United States and Europe. This system is uncomplicated, but has proven to be inefficient and cumbersome.

In this system, as the dentist begins the examination in the upper right quadrant at the location of the third molar, each tooth is numbered from 1 to 32 (in the adult dentition) proceeding in a clockwise direction from that point. The maxillary right third molar is tooth no. 1 and, continuing around to the mandibular right side, the third molar is tooth no. 32.

This system helps you remember the numbers contained in each quadrant, but it is not as efficient as the International system. The maxillary right quadrant contains numbers 1 to 8, the maxillary left quadrant contains numbers 9 to 16, the mandibular left quadrant contains numbers 17 to 24, and the mandibular right quadrant contains numbers 25 to 32. A problem can occur if a tooth is extracted and the adjacent tooth drifts into that position. This makes identification difficult. Also, many adults do not have all four third molars, and this, too, impedes the process of identification.

In the Universal Tooth Numbering System, the primary teeth are identified by letters instead of numbers. Beginning at the maxillary right second primary molar and continuing in a clockwise direction, the first tooth is identified with the letter A. The next molar is B, the cuspid is C, the lateral is D, and the incisor is E.

It helps to memorize the range of letters within each quadrant.

Maxillary right contains letters A to E.

Maxillary left contains letters F to J.

Mandibular left contains letters K to O.

Mandibular right contains letters P to T.

This identification system works well when the quadrants are memorized and the teeth are counted. However, problems can occur when teeth drift from their normal position or are congenitally missing.

EXHIBIT 5.6 UNIVERSAL TOOTH NUMBERING SYSTEM: ADULT DENTITION

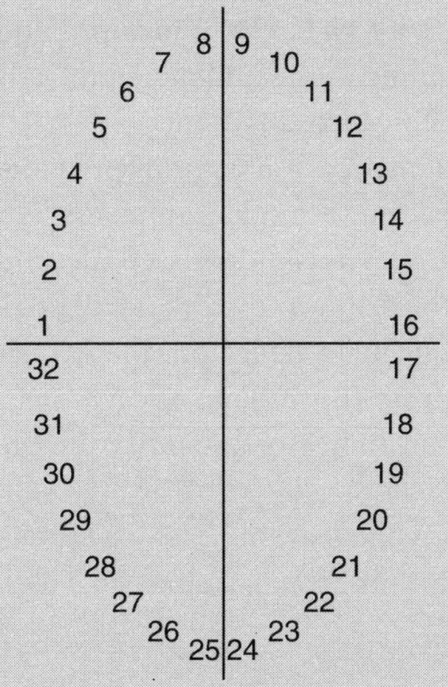

EXHIBIT 5.7 UNIVERSAL TOOTH NUMBERING SYSTEM: PRIMARY DENTITION

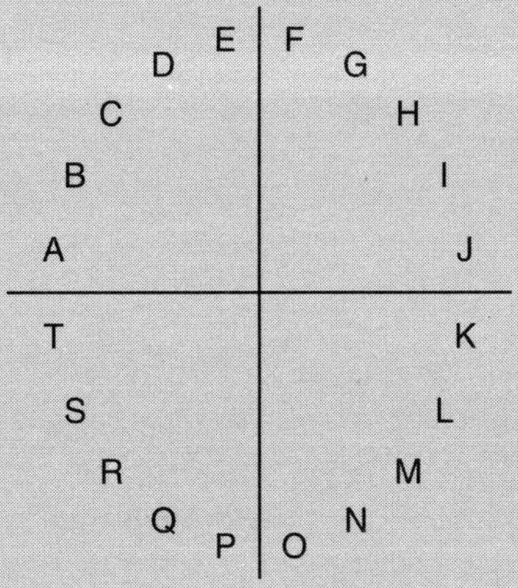

PALMER'S IDENTIFICATION SYSTEM

The Palmer's system of tooth identification presents a more graphic illustration of where the tooth is located in each quadrant. This system uses a symbol to indicate the quadrant.

It is helpful to think of the vertical line as the midline and the horizontal line as the transverse plane. These boxes enclose the tooth number in such a way that the quadrant and the tooth number are identified. Beginning at the midline, in the adult dentition, the teeth are numbered 1 to 8 in each quadrant.

Palmer's Identification System provides an efficient method of instant identification through graphic representation of the tooth location. Just as the previously discussed identification systems differentiated between the adult and primary dentition, so does the Palmer's system. For the primary dentition, the Palmer's system uses lower case letters starting from the midline of each quadrant. These letters, along with the quadrant indicators, identify the precise location and type of tooth.

It is helpful while learning each of these systems to practise counting your own teeth in front of a mirror. This will simulate looking into

EXHIBIT 5.8 **MIDSAGITTAL PLANE**

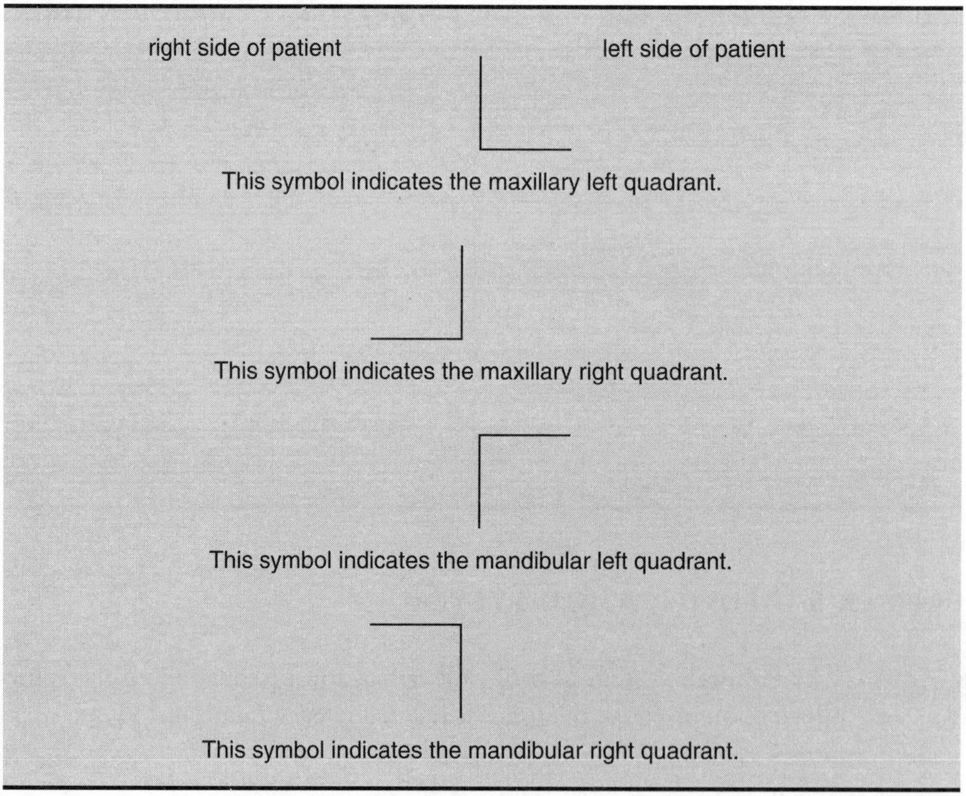

right side of patient   left side of patient

This symbol indicates the maxillary left quadrant.

This symbol indicates the maxillary right quadrant.

This symbol indicates the mandibular left quadrant.

This symbol indicates the mandibular right quadrant.

EXHIBIT 5.9 PALMER'S IDENTIFICATION SYSTEM: ADULT DENTITION

1⌐

This indicates that the tooth is the mandibular left central incisor.

⌐6

This indicates that the tooth is the maxillary right first molar (6 year).

4, 5⌐

This represents the maxillary left first and second bicuspid.

EXHIBIT 5.10 PALMER'S IDENTIFICATION SYSTEM: PRIMARY DENTITION

right side of patient   left side of patient

abcde⌐

This indicates all of the teeth in the
maxillary left quadrant of the primary dentition.

⌐edcba

This indicates all of the teeth in the
maxillary right quadrant of the primary dentiton.

abcde⌐

This indicates all of the teeth in the
mandibular left quadrant of the primary dentition.

⌐edcba

This indicates all of the teeth in the
mandibular right quadrant of the primary dentiton.

a patient's mouth. Count out loud (if possible) while using your fore-finger against your teeth to identify the teeth. It is even more helpful if you can ask friends or family members to allow you to identify their teeth. Try to also identify the restorations.

ASSIGNMENT

1. a. How many systems are there to identify teeth by numbers?
   b. What are the names of the tooth numbering systems?
2. How many teeth are there in the permanent dentition?
3. How many teeth are there in the primary dentition?
4. According to the International Tooth Numbering System, identify the following teeth:
   a. the mandibular right 6-year molar _____
   b. the maxillary right central incisor _____
   c. the maxillary left first bicuspid _____
   d. the mandibular left lateral incisor _____
5. According to the International Tooth Numbering System, describe the location of the following teeth: (e.g., 2.6 = maxillary left first molar):
   a. 1.7 _____
   b. 3.8 _____
   c. 4.3 _____
   d. 5.4 _____
6. According to the Universal Tooth Numbering System, identify the following teeth:
   a. the mandibular right 6-year molar _____
   b. the maxillary right central incisor _____
   c. the maxillary left first bicuspid _____
   d. the mandibular left lateral incisor _____
   e. the mandibular left wisdom tooth _____

7. Identify the following teeth according to Palmer's Identification System.

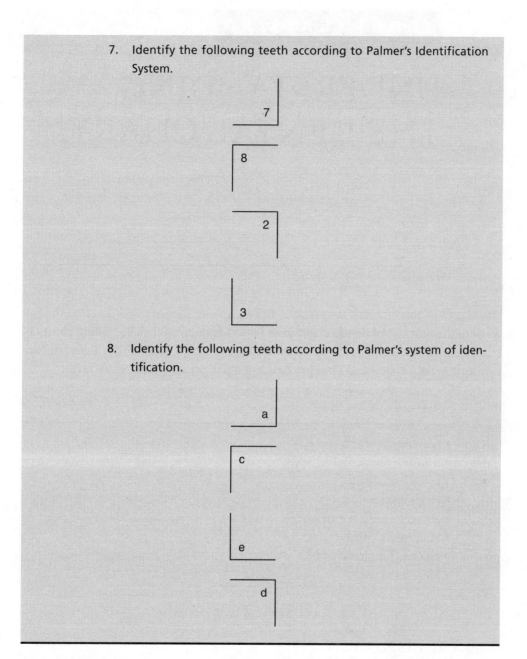

8. Identify the following teeth according to Palmer's system of identification.

CHAPTER SIX

UNDERSTANDING THE DENTAL CHART

OBJECTIVE

At the end of this chapter, the student will be able to identify and describe the following: the purpose of dental charts, the reason for accuracy in recording chart entries, how to recognize and record medical alerts, how to record a three-surface restoration on a chart, and how to complete a patient medical history form.

TOPICS

- patient medical history
- transferring dental records
- confidentiality
- chart entries
- correcting chart entries
- reading a dental chart
- colour coding a chart
- medical alerts

MEDICAL HISTORIES

A complete medical history must be obtained from new patients. This detailed information is necessary to help the dentist evaluate the patient's physical condition, including any special treatment considerations. (See Exhibit 6.1 for an example of a medical history chart.) It is essential for the medical history to be accurate, legible, and complete. Many dental office administrators will help the patient complete a health questionnaire. Some dentists prefer to ask the patient the health

EXHIBIT 6.1   MEDICAL HISTORY FORM

Last Name:	First	Middle

Please ✔ YES or NO to each question. If unsure of a question, please consult with the dentist. YES NO

1. Are you being treated for any medical condition at present or within the past two years? If yes, please explain:
   _____ Physician: _____ Phone: _____
2. Have you been hospitalized in the past two years? _____
3. When was your last visit to a Physician? _____ Last complete physical examination? _____
4. Have you recently, or are you presently, taking any PRESCRIPTION or NON-PRESCRIPTION drugs? Please list:
   1. _____ 2. _____ 3. _____
   4. _____ 5. _____ 6. _____
5. Have you ever reacted adversely to any of the following? (Please circle.) ANTIBIOTICS - Penicillin, Sulfonamide, other antibiotics, ASPIRIN, BARBITURATES (sleeping pills), CODEINE, DARVON, LOCAL ANAESTHETIC (freezing), NITROUS OXIDE, any other medicine: _____
6. Have you ever been advised against taking any specific type of medication? _____
7. Do you have any of the following? Asthma, Hay Fever, Food Allergies, Metal or Latex Allergies, Skin Rashes, Hives, or any other allergic conditions?
8. Do any of these allergic conditions result in headache, nausea, swelling, shortness of breath, or chest constriction? If so, please explain: _____
9. Has any family member had diabetes? _____
10. Do you bleed EXCESSIVELY from a cut or injury, or bruise easily? _____
11. Do your ankles, feet or hands swell? _____
12. Has your weight, appetite or energy level changed dramatically recently? _____
13. Do you experience shortness of breath or chest pain when taking a walk or climbing stairs? _____
14. Do you follow a special diet? _____
15. Have you tested HIV positive? _____
16. Do you have FREQUENT SEVERE headaches, earaches, ear/throat infections? _____
17. Have you ever had any injury or surgery to your face or jaws? _____
18. Do you wear eyeglasses or contact lenses? _____
19. Do you have any hearing difficulties? _____
20. Do you smoke or use any other forms of tobacco? _____
    Are you wearing the transdermal nicotine patch? _____
21. Are you alcohol and/or drug dependent? _____
    and, Have you received treatment? _____
22. INDICATE WHICH OF THE FOLLOWING YOU PRESENTLY HAVE OR EVER HAD:

	YES NO		YES NO		YES NO
A.I.D.S.	☐	Head/neck injuries	☐	Malignant Hyperthermia	☐
Anemia	☐	Heart disease or attack	☐	Mental/nervous disorder	☐
Angina pectoris	☐	Heart murmur	☐	Mitral valve prolapse	☐
Arthritis/rheumatism	☐	Heart pacemaker	☐	Organ transplant/medical implant	☐
Artificial heart valve	☐	Heart rhythm disorder	☐	Psychiatric treatment	☐
Artificial joints(hip, knee)	☐	Heart surgery	☐	Radiation treatment/chemotherapy	☐
Blood disorders	☐	Hepatitis A	☐	Rheumatic/Scarlet fever	☐
Bronchitis	☐	Hepatitis B	☐	Sickle cell disease	☐
Cancer	☐	Hepatitis C	☐	Sinus trouble	☐
Circulation problems	☐	Herpes	☐	Stomach/intestinal problems	☐
Congenital heart lesions	☐	High/Low blood pressure	☐	Stroke	☐
Cortisone/steroid	☐	Hodgkins disease	☐	Thyroid disease	☐
Diabetes	☐	Hyper (Hypo) Glycemia	☐	Tuberculosis	☐
Emphysema	☐	Hypertension	☐	Ulcers	☐
Epilepsy or seizures	☐	Jaundice	☐	Venereal Disease	☐
Fainting or dizzy spells	☐	Kidney disease	☐	Other _____	☐
Glandular disorders	☐	Liver disease	☐	Other _____	☐
Glaucoma	☐	Lung disease	☐	Other _____	☐

23. Has the CHILD PATIENT recently had any of the following: (indicate approximate date.)	Measles _____ Mumps _____ Chicken Pox _____		Strep throat _____ Tonsillitis _____	

24. WOMEN ONLY: Are you pregnant or suspect you may be? _____
    If yes, what is the expected delivery date? _____ Are you taking any birth control pills? _____

25. Do you currently have, or have you had in the past, any disease, condition or problem not listed above? _____
26. Is there anything else about your health we should be made aware of? _____
27. Do you wish to speak to the Doctor privately about any problem or medical condition? _____

The DMD (Dental Management Document) and the DMD Emergency Treatment System have been reproduced with the permission of Dental Risk Management Systems Inc., which holds the copyright.

history questions when the patient is in the dental chair. A patient's health history should be reviewed at every appointment for any changes.

An accurate and complete medical history will provide the patient with optimum care and the dental office with legal protection against legal action. Regardless of whether the patient completes his or her own health questionnaire or it is completed with the assistance of a staff member, it is necessary to respect the **patient's right to privacy**. A patient's medical history should not be discussed in the presence of other patients. Some questions may be embarrassing. Patients will usually provide honest and complete answers if they feel comfortable and assured that their right to privacy is being preserved and protected.

The general information area on a new patient form will include the full name, address, city, postal code, and telephone number. If the patient does not mind being called at work, you can obtain the work telephone number as well.

Chart entries should always be made in ink. To make a correction in a chart, cross through the error and initial it. Never use correction fluid in a dental chart. Remember, the dental chart is a legal document.

A thorough medical history should include any childhood illnesses, current medications, and contagious diseases such as hepatitis, allergies, heart problems, etc. Health alerts should be noted in *red* on the front of the patient's chart, inside the chart, and on the chart cover. Red is the international symbol for health alert. A code may be used, such as HA for Health Alert or MA for Medical Alert. This will draw the attention of the dentist, who will obtain the necessary medical details before commencing treatment.

Health Alerts

A patient may be allergic to medications, such as anaesthetics. Dentists often prescribe antibiotics or analgesic medications, which could lead to an allergic reaction or even anaphylactic shock if the allergy is not made known to the dentist.

Contagious illnesses (e.g., hepatitis B, tuberculosis, or AIDS) can endanger dental care providers and other patients. Discretion and tact should be exercised when obtaining sensitive information from patients and when recording it on dental charts.

Heart problems, past and present (e.g., rheumatic fever, pacemaker implant, mitral valve prolapse, heart murmur) should be indicated. Most dental procedures involve some bleeding, even though it may be minimal. If the patient has an existing heart condition, bacteria from the mouth can enter the bloodstream and cause a dangerous condition called endocarditis, which affects the valves within the heart.

A patient with a pacemaker implanted should not be near ultrasonic equipment (e.g., sterilizers) because it could cause an irregular signal to the pacemaker, resulting in an arrhythmia (irregular heart beat).

Hereditary factors should be considered. For example, diabetes and heart disease are both considered to have hereditary links. Patients who suffer from arthritis may be taking Aspirin or other types of anti-inflammatory drugs. These drugs also act as anticoagulants, or blood thinners, and can cause excessive bleeding during dental procedures. The dentist should be alerted to patients who are taking anti-inflammatory drugs of any kind.

Previous dental experiences are important for the doctor to be aware of. A patient who has had a negative experience in the past will tend to be nervous and anxious. The dental team should offer reassurance and help the patient relax before seeing the dentist. A relaxed patient responds well to treatment, and this enhances the recovery process. For someone with a cardiac history, anxiety before dental treatment can cause potential health hazards. All dental staff should be trained in emergency procedures and cardiopulmonary resuscitation (CPR).

PURPOSES OF THE DENTAL CHART

A clinical record of treatment is kept on every patient. The clinical record is called the chart. The dental office administrator is responsible for the care and control of the clinical records in a dental practice. Although the dental care providers will be making most of the handwritten entries in the chart, the administrator must be able to read the chart in order to extract important information that is needed for administration purposes.

Why is the clinical record so important? The purpose of the clinical record is to assist in the diagnosis and treatment of the patient. It is necessary for the dental provider to know as much as possible about the patient's past experience along with the medical and dental history of the patient.

The chart should be accurate, legible, and complete, to comply with laws and provide legal protection for the dentist as well as to ensure that the patient is receiving appropriate dental care.

A standard method for charting is represented by the acronym SOAP. This represents

Subjective information—symptoms, what the patient feels

Objective information—what the dentist observes

Assessment—the diagnosis reached from the subjective and objective information

Plan—the treatment plan and probable outcome

The chart serves as a record of the diagnosis and treatment plan. The diagnosis is reached after the dentist has received subjective information from the patient, or what the patient feels, along with additional information. The dentist will also record objective information, or what is observed on examination. The examination will usually include diagnostic aids such as x-rays and tests. A combination of the subjective and objective information will assist the dentist in making an accurate assessment of the patient's dental health. A comprehensive treatment plan will then be prepared to bring the patient to optimal dental health.

A complete oral diagnosis and treatment plan will usually consist of three alternative levels of treatment. The first choice will be the treatment plan that will restore the teeth to optimal function and aesthetics. This will include an ongoing preventive care program and may incorporate the use of precious metals in the restorative procedures.

The second level of treatment would be a standard care program. This treatment will provide the restoration of function, and use of semi-precious metals, amalgam, removable prostheses, etc. may be indicated. A standard dental care program will also include a preventive care program.

An emergency care level of treatment will provide the patient with relief of a painful condition. This plan does not usually include preventive maintenance care.

All patient information is **highly confidential,** whether it concerns a patient's medical or financial information. It is the responsibility of all staff members to secure each patient's right to privacy. If confidential medical information is released by an employee, the dentist is held responsible under the doctrine of *respondent superior* or "let the master answer." The employee, however, is still responsible for his or her own actions, and the injured party may file suit against the dental office staff member.

Charts should be locked in a fireproof cabinet when the office is closed. They should also always be kept away from the view of other patients. Caution should be exercised when holding conversations within the office or over the telephone regarding a patient's confidential information.

Is the chart the property of the patient or the dentist?

The chart is the legal property of the dentist. The dentist is responsible for producing and securing it. The chart is also a legal document and is admissible in court in the case of a malpractice suit. Forensic dental pathologists may require the clinical chart to identify a person who has been disfigured or had died. Third party insurance carriers may require an audit of a clinical chart by one of their dental consultants. Maintaining and updating the clinical charts is the responsibility of the dentist as well as the dental office administrator with the cooperation of the entire dental team.

Transferring Patient Records

A patient may ask to take his or her chart when transferring to another dental office. For the legal protection of the dentist, it is necessary to obtain a written consent from the patient before transferring the records to anyone. The clinical record may then be copied and forwarded to the receiving office. The dentist should keep the original chart along with the original signed consent from the patient. X-rays can be copied and forwarded with the copied chart if the office has an x-ray duplicator. In most cases, if recent x-rays were taken, they will be forwarded to the new dental office to prevent subjecting the patient to unnecessary radiation exposure.

Because transferring records by mail may be risky, a courier service is recommended. The administrator should retain the receipt from the courier service verifying the transfer. A fee can be charged to the patient to cover costs associated with the transfer of records.

CHARTING

During the clinical examination, the dentist identifies pathologic conditions and dictates the findings to an assistant. The assistant will then record the findings on the patient's clinical record. The dentist or the assistant may follow a specific method for charting the dental conditions present and this method will vary from office to office. It is important to be consistent with charting symbols and ensure that all staff are aware of what the symbols represent.

Charting symbols are used to present a visual picture of the restoration or dental condition. Although the office administrator will not be responsible for charting actual dental conditions, it will be most helpful to know how to read the clinical chart. Dental professionals occasionally write down an incorrect tooth number on a communication slip; this can be checked on the chart. Most dental charts will provide a method of charting on all three views of the tooth: the facial view, the lingual view, and the occlusal view.

The facial view is how the tooth appears when viewed from a frontal perspective. The facial surfaces touch the lips (anteriorly) and the cheeks (posteriorly).

The lingual view is how the tooth appears from the tongue. The dentist looks at the back surface of the tooth that touches the tongue.

The occlusal view represents tooth surfaces from the lateral plane, which runs across the occlusal and incisal surfaces.

Representations of all three views of the teeth are necessary to record information about three-dimensional objects (teeth) accurately onto a one-dimensional plane.

There are so many variations in dental charting that it would be an arduous task to identify all of the charting symbols that are used. Standardization of charting symbols would be helpful, but there are too many differences between offices. For example, in some systems an X is used to indicate a missing tooth. In other systems a single slash (/) is used for this purpose. A colour coding system may be used to indicate restorations and defects. If the condition noted requires future treatment, it may be charted in red, whereas an existing condition may be charted in blue. Charting pencils with blue on one end and red on the opposite end have been designed for this purpose.

The following are examples of some commonly used colour codes:

- Carious lesions are outlined on the tooth surface in pencil; for example, a mesio-occlusal cavity would be outlined on the facial and occlusal surfaces.
- When the tooth is restored, the area is filled in with the appropriate colour.
- Amalgam restorations are filled in on the tooth surfaces in blue.
- Composite restorations may be shaded in green to show the difference in restorative material.

TABLE 6.1 **COMMON CHARTING SYMBOLS**

Am	amalgam filling
Au	gold
E	
Ext.	extraction
Incip.	incipient caries, or decay that has not yet penetrated the enamel
Er	erosion
RCT	root canal therapy
PJC	porcelain jacket crown
PFM	porcelain fused to metal crown
Ab	abrasion
⬜	(around a tooth) a missing tooth
◯	(red circle around the apex of the root) an abscessed tooth
red dots	incipient caries
blue vertical line from crown to apex	root canal therapy completed

• If the restored tooth needs a new restoration, the pertinent area is outlined in the colour corresponding to the colour of the intended restoration.

Note that when submitting a predetermination for a bridge, it is advisable to ask the patient when the tooth or teeth were extracted. Since many patients will have difficulty remembering the exact date, an approximate date or year will be acceptable. The insurance company will require that information to see if the claim is eligible for the missing tooth exclusion. Refer to Chapter 7 for more information.

EXHIBIT 6.2 **DENTAL CHART**

The DMD (Dental Management Document) and the DMD Emergency Treatment System have been reproduced with the permission of Dental Risk Management Systems Inc., which holds the copyright.

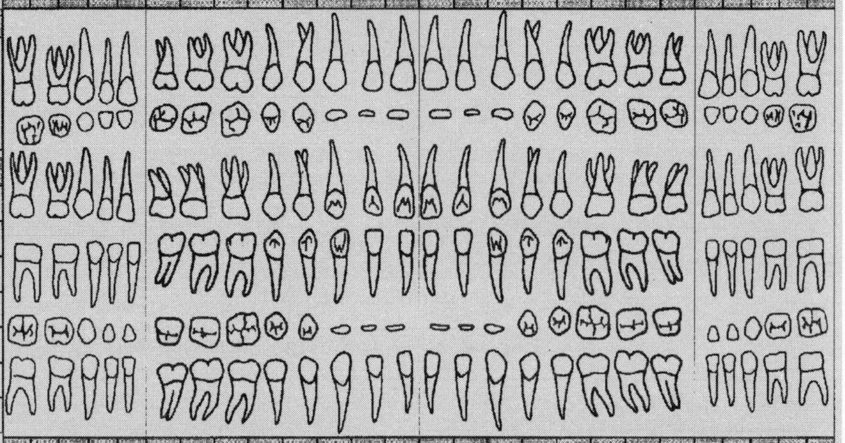

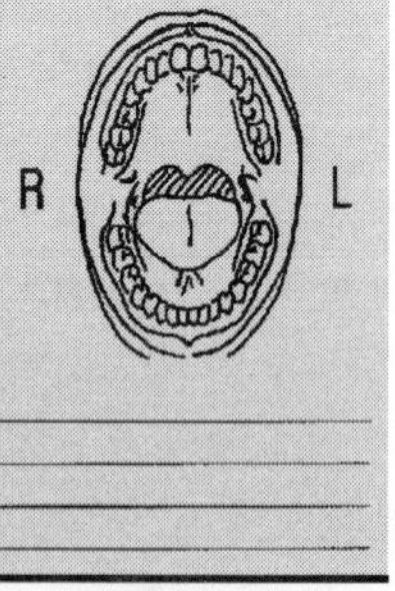

ASSIGNMENT

On the chart below, identify the conditions present. Assume that all conditions are existing.

The DMD (Dental Management Document) and the DMD Emergency Treatment System have been reproduced with the permission of Dental Risk Management Systems Inc., which holds the copyright.

Example: tooth no. 1.8   MO amalgam

_____   _____

_____   _____

_____   _____

_____   _____

_____   _____

_____   _____

_____   _____

_____   _____

Answers

Tooth no. 1.8 – MO amalgam

Tooth no. 1.6 – gold crown

Tooth no. 1.3 – root canal therapy

Tooth no. 1.1 – incipient caries on the labial surface

Tooth no. 2.3 – missing

Tooth no. 2.6 – requires extraction

Tooth no. 2.7 – MOD amalgam

Tooth no. 3.8 – impacted wisdom tooth

Tooth no. 3.4 – Li. Occ. amalgam

Tooth no. 4.3 – 3 mm periodontal pockets

Teeth nos. 4.6, 4.7, 4.8 – a three-unit bridge.

Tooth no 4.7 is missing, therefore, it is the pontic.

Teeth nos. 4.6 and 4.8 are the abutment teeth.

CHAPTER SEVEN

DENTAL INSURANCE

OBJECTIVE

At the end of this chapter, the student will be able to identify and describe the following: categories of dental services, components of a dental insurance claim form, methods of assisting patients in understanding their insurance programs, and types of insurance programs available.

TOPICS

- definition of insurance
- types of insurance programs
- coordination of benefits
- the role of the office administrator
- understanding the fee guide
- categories of service
- components of an insurance form
- completing insurance forms
- predeterminations

WHAT IS INSURANCE?

Insurance programs provide protection against financial loss. People who wish to be insured will purchase a contract from an insuring company to protect what they feel is of value to them. The person who purchases the contract is known as the insured. For example, life insurance is purchased to provide financial protection to the next of kin should the insured person die. Car insurance is purchased to provide protection to the car owner in the event of a costly accident.

The company that designs and sells the insurance contract is known as the insurer. The insurance company can also be known as the carrier because it is carrying the policy and assuming the financial risk.

Dental insurance operates on the same basic concept as other types of insurance, except that it is usually designed and administered under a group contract. Group insurance simply means that a particular company may purchase an insurance contract for the group of employees who work at that company. The company will negotiate the design and cost of the specific plan with the insurance carrier. The plan design will determine how much coverage the employees will receive.

For example, if a company such as General Motors decides to provide its employees with a dental plan as part of a benefits package, it would then contact an insurance company, such as Canada Life Insurance Company, Great West Life Assurance Co., or any of several that can provide group insurance coverage. The insurance company would then design a program that meets the specific needs of the employees of General Motors.

The group insurance representative would discuss with the plan administrator for General Motors how much the policy will cost and how much coverage it will provide. The fee structure for the plan would be based on a statistical analysis of the insured group that would include an estimate of how many claims the insurance company might expect to pay.

Once the insurance program is agreed upon, the insurance contract is offered to the employees. An employee who decides to subscribe to the insurance program will then apply for benefits through the employer.

The employee who has subscribed is now called the subscriber or *guarantor*. Insurance programs are essentially a contract between the employee and the insurance carrier, not between the insurance carrier and the dentist.

Eligibility Requirements

Most group insurance programs have a specific requirement that the insured party (employee) has been with the company for at least 90 days, and in some cases one year. This reduces the risk of the employee simply taking advantage of the dental plan and then dropping out of the program or leaving the job—a process called antiselection or selection against the insurer. When this occurs, the amount of risk increases for the insuring company, who therefore may need to increase the premiums. It is because of increased premiums that many companies have drastically reduced the coverage that is offered and in some cases have eliminated dental programs altogether.

An employee who joins the dental plan can apply for single or family coverage. When an employee selects family coverage, all family members are eligible for insured dental care. The employee's family then become the eligible members or dependants.

When the guarantor or his or her family member goes to the dentist, the dentist charges a fee for the services rendered. The guarantor (employee) pays the fee to the dentist and then submits an insurance form to the carrier in order to receive some or all of the money back.

This type of contract is called an *indemnity* contract. Indemnity is defined as that which is given as compensation for loss or damage. With this type of contract, the claims are paid as benefits are used.

Assignment of Benefits

Insurance benefits belong to the person who is insured. Therefore, the insured patient is responsible for payment to the dentist and is subsequently reimbursed by the insurance carrier according to the contract that was purchased.

The contract of insurance is between the insured and the carrier, and the *beneficiary* is usually the insured. The patient may, however, assign the benefit to the dentist. The insurance company will then pay the claim to the dentist directly. This is called accepting assignment or assignment of claims. In this case, the insured assigns a beneficiary (the dentist), thus relinquishing the right to accept the payment for that particular claim. Most dental offices throughout Canada do not encourage assignment of claims.

CAPITATION PROGRAM

In capitation, a company will purchase a group insurance contract at a reduced cost, on condition that all of the employees insured under it attend specified dental offices. The insurance company will approach dentists within the community to perform services on these groups of employees for a cost per capita. This concept is also known as a prepaid insurance program. The dentist who is involved in a prepaid dental program will receive a payment each month based on the number of members who have selected that dental office.

For example, if a company has 100 employees who are part of a capitation program, the carrier may have contracted with five dentists to provide services for the employees. In return, the insurance company will pay each dentist a fee per month, whether or not the patient attends the office for dental care. Controversy exists as to whether there is sufficient incentive for the dental services provider to administer appropriate care for the patient in such programs. In fact, some people believe that it may encourage providers to administer less than optimal treatment.

A capitation concept, as presented here, will restrict the patient's freedom of choice for dental care. Those who wish to be provided with insured dental treatment must attend one of the dentists chosen by the insurance company. This concept is common in the medical community and is known as Health Management Organization (HMO). This approach to health care delivery is very popular in the United States.

Insurance companies do not dictate treatment to patients. However, patients generally feel that if an insurance company will not cover a service, then it is assumed to be unnecessary.

PREFERRED PROVIDER ORGANIZATION

Another form of insurance contract is a Preferred Provider Organization (PPO). In this case, dentists—the preferred providers—are contracted by the insurance carrier to work under a *fixed fee schedule* to provide services to a specific group.

For example, employees under a PPO contract are given a choice of several dental offices. However, if they choose to attend a dentist outside the group, coverage will be limited to the amount designated for services at the reduced fee. This is similar to a standard indemnity contract, except for the providers agreeing to work for discounted fees for that particular group.

SHARED RISK

To prevent abuse of insurance contract benefits, carriers will sometimes require that patients have some vested interest in their dental health care through the use of *copayments*.

If a patient has a dental plan that will pay 80 percent of the cost of dental care and the patient is responsible for 20 percent, the 20 percent is called the copayment. The patient is assuming 20 percent of the responsibility for his or her own care, thus reducing the risk to the carrier from procedures that are unnecessary. Insurance carriers are concerned with the overuse of dental benefits, which increase the cost of programs to employers.

When patients become informed consumers they share the responsibility of determining how their health care dollars are directed. When a patient shares in the financial responsibility of their health care, the cost of the insurance program is usually reduced by informed and wise choices for treatment.

A subscriber may also be required to share responsibility through the use of a deductible. Just as with car insurance, when a dental claim is made, the patient may have to pay the first $25 before the insurance coverage takes effect. This is usually an annual deductible, which can be based on the calendar year or the contract year. An example of a typical group dental insurance program is as follows:

80 percent coverage for routine services

60 percent for major restorative services

50 percent for orthodontic services

a $25 annual deductible

Routine care is usually considered to include services that would provide maintenance and preservation of the oral structure. These would include prophylaxis and scaling, fillings, and root canal therapy, as well as diagnostic services such as radiographs, study casts, and biopsies.

Major restorative services consist of crowns, bridges, dentures, etc. This category may include periodontal surgery and complex oral surgery. A patient copayment is always included in the dental insurance plan for these services.

Orthodontic services are those which involve alignment of the jaw and straightening of teeth. Many children aged 12 or more may require orthodontic treatment and, in fact, it is now fashionable for adults to pursue orthodontic correction. This benefit can become very expensive and is often not included in insurance contracts.

Dental insurance programs are very costly to employers and/or to individuals because they are considered to be a "living" benefit. In other words, a life insurance claim is paid only when the insured party dies, and a single payment is made, whereas dental insurance claims are paid on a regular basis because people who purchase the insurance generally use their benefits. This pattern of utilization is known to an insurance company as claims experience.

EXCLUSIONS AND LIMITATIONS

To reduce the amount of claims experience on a particular program, many insurance contracts will include an **exclusions and/or limitations clause.** An example of this common clause is the missing tooth exclusion. What this means is that if the subscriber to the insurance program has a pre-existing condition, such as a missing tooth, then replacement of that tooth through fixed or removable prosthodontics is excluded from the contract. Cosmetic dentistry and orthodontics are frequent exclusions from dental contracts.

Some insurance contracts may provide coverage for treatment of pre-existing conditions but limit the amount of coverage through an **alternate benefits clause.** For example, if a patient with missing teeth requires a three-unit bridge on anterior teeth, at an estimated cost of $1,500, the insurance company may state that the contract will cover the amount of an alternate benefit. In other words, what it will cover would be the amount of a partial denture, approximately $250. Please note that this does not indicate that the insurance company is dictating the treatment of choice, or implying that the partial denture is a preferred treatment over a three-unit bridge. It is simply stating that the amount of financial reimbursement is limited to $250.

Another example of a limitation is the six- or nine-month recall appointment. Recall appointments are necessary to preventive dental care; however, the insurance companies may limit their frequency as part of the contract design. Some programs provide for a six-month recall but cover the cost of bite-wing x-rays to be taken only once per year.

The dental office administrator should be very aware of the limitations of insurance programs, particularly when scheduling recall appointments. For example, a patient treated one day before the six-month period is completed will not be eligible for reimbursement. It is the administrator's responsibility to make sure that the patient's appointment is scheduled at the appropriate time. Remember, when scheduling recall appointments, **to check the date of the last recall first.**

Exclusions and limitations are very important concepts for the dental office administrator to understand and to be able to discuss comfortably with patients. Unfortunately, insurance coverage does affect the patient's decision-making process, but a professional dental office administrator can help the patient make an informed choice based on the facts and the dentist's recommendations for treatment. Most patients will select high quality dental care over alternate benefits if they truly understand the reason for the treatment of choice.

It is important for the dental office administrator to realize that the insurance program design is unique to each employer or individual who has purchased the insurance. Assisting patients to understand and gain full benefit from their insurance program is an important aspect of your overall success as a dental office administrator. It is helpful to indicate the necessary information regarding the patient's insurance on the chart or perhaps the ledger card.

Here is an example:

100 R

50 M

50 O

current

Blue Cross, subscriber—Mr. Smith

This will indicate that the patient is covered 100 percent for routine care (based on the current fee guide), 50 percent for major restorative services, and 50 percent for orthodontic care. This chart or ledger entry will be helpful when completing predeterminations and insurance forms.

When new patients call, the dental office administrator should ask if they have insurance and direct them to bring any necessary information to the first appointment. This allows you an opportunity to help them fill out their forms and understand their benefits. During new patient interviews, the dental office administrator can educate new patients on the financial procedures and payment policies of the practice.

PREDETERMINATION OF BENEFITS

Prior to the provision of dental services, most insurance contracts require a predetermination to be submitted to the insurance company for all comprehensive treatment. The insurance company will require all relevant radiographs and any further necessary information relating to the case. For example, they may require the date the tooth was extracted for a crown and bridge predetermination, to determine whether this complies with the missing tooth exclusion clause.

When the insurance company approves payment for the recommended procedure, treatment may be started. Approval will be sent to the subscriber (insured) along with a copy to the dental office. If this procedure is not followed correctly, the insurance company has the right to refuse to cover the cost of the services, leaving the patient solely responsible for the cost.

It is important for the dental office administrator to note that this process generally takes four to six weeks. At the time of the initial consultation, the patient understands the reason for the treatment and is psychologically prepared to "buy" the treatment. The time delay may cause the patient to change his or her mind regarding the treatment. Insurance companies depend on this psychological phenomenon in an effort to keep claims to a minimum.

It is crucial for the dental office administrator to follow up with the patient during this time. This helps the patient to realize the necessity for the treatment and it lets the patient know that the dental care provider cares about him or her. Effective follow-up will also help the dental office administrator to control the financial productivity of the practice. Every predetermination that has been sent and not followed up represents lost revenue for the practice. Proper completion of forms is essential; however, follow-up is more important. Each predetermination that has been sent should be filed by order of date in a binder. When confirmation has been received, the patient should be called to make an appointment.

Insurance companies usually require radiographs. **Radiographs are the property of the dentist** as they are taken for diagnostic purposes. However, many dentists will allow them to be released from the practice for the purpose of predetermination. If the office has an x-ray duplicator, the ideal situation would be to send the duplicate x-rays. If not, then the x-rays should be labelled with the name of the patient and the name and address of the dental office. Intra-oral cameras and computers will eventually be helpful tools for dental offices in predetermination procedures and the adjudication of claims.

COORDINATION OF BENEFITS

The purpose of a **coordination of benefits clause** is to prevent duplication of benefits. Many Canadian families now have two or more

EXHIBIT 7.1 PREDETERMINATION FORM

STANDARD DENTAL PRE-TREATMENT FORM

Approved by the Ontario Dental Association

	DATE PREPARED			THIS ESTIMATE IS VALID UNTIL		
	DAY	MO	YEAR	DAY	MO	YEAR
	29	11	96	28	02	97

UNIQUE NO. **0687752**   SPEC.   PATIENT'S OFFICE ACCOUNT NO. **03224**

PATIENT

LAST NAME **Walker, Mr.** GIVEN NAME **Johnny A.**

ADDRESS **235 Main St. E.** APT

CITY **Hamilton, ON** PROV. POSTAL CODE **L0H 1T0**

DENTIST

John Hollis, B.A., D.D.S.
650 Maple Road
Burlington, ON L7M 7H4
PHONE NO. **(905) 333-3200**

DENTIST'S SIGNATURE

ADDITIONAL COMMENTS: Use this space to provide additional information or description pertinent to the treatment plan.

Examination: (Fees Only)	$	
Radiographs: (Fees Only)	$	
Other Diagnostic Service: (Total Fee Only)	$	+L
Oral Hygiene Instructions: (Fee Only)	$	
Other Preventive Services:	$	
Prophylaxis/fluoride: (Fee Only)	$	
Basic Restorative Services: Do not itemize surfaces, fees or teeth here. (Total Fee Only)	$	
Surgery: (Total Fee Only)	$	+L
Periodontal Services: (Total Fee Only)	$ **683.00**	+L
Endodontic Services: Tooth	$	
(Give Fee per Tooth) Tooth	$	
Tooth	$	
Tooth	$	
Tooth	$	
Tooth	$	
Anaesthetic Services: (Total Fee Only)	$	+Drugs
Orthodontic Services: (Total Fee Only)	$	+L

Other Services including Crowns, Bridges, Dentures: Itemize tooth, service, professional fee but not commercial lab charge.

26 27211 Porcelain Fused to Metal C	$ **475.00**	+L
	$	+L
	$	+L
	$	+L
	$	+L
	$	+L
	$	+L
	$	+L
	$	+L
	$	+L

Total Estimated Lab Charges $ **200.00**

TOTAL ESTIMATE $ **1358.00**

THIS SECTION TO BE COMPLETED BY PATIENT

SUBSCRIBER

NAME **Johnny A. Walker**

ADDRESS **235 Main St. E.**
Hamilton, ON   L0H 1T0

EMPLOYER **ABEL Computers Ltd.**

ADDRESS

GROUP POLICY	CERTIFICATE NO.	SOC. INS. NO.
35634	**4343343**	

PATIENT'S DATE OF BIRTH

DAY	MTH	YEAR	RELATIONSHIP TO SUBSCRIBER
03	03	36	

I authorize the release of the information outlined in this treatment form to my insuring company or its agents.

SIGNATURE OF PATIENT (OR GUARDIA/ I/PARENT)

L IS AN APPROXIMATION ONLY. FINAL LABORATORY CHARGES WILL BE INCLUDED ON CLAIM FORM.

H SERVICES MARKED (H) WILL BE PERFORMED IN HOSPITAL.

Revision 85.3 (oct/85)

Sample provided by ABEL Computers Ltd., Burlington, Ontario.

family members who are eligible for dental benefits through their employers. This can cause duplication of coverage and can encourage the insured parties to select the insurance program that provides the most coverage. To give insurance companies protection against antiselection and to provide the patient with an efficient claims adjudication process, it is helpful for the dental office administrator to be familiar with how coordination of benefits (COB) is administered.

If the insured members are covered for family benefits under more than one insurance plan, then it is essential to determine which is the primary carrier and which is the secondary carrier. The primary carrier is the insurance company that is responsible for first payment of the claim. This is always the company to which the patient is a subscriber.

For example, Mr. and Mrs. Smith work at separate companies, both with dental insurance coverage through their employer. Mr. Smith works at General Motors and is insured by Great West Life. Mrs. Smith works at Sears and is insured by Canada Life. When Mr. Smith goes to the dentist, his carrier, Great West Life, is automatically the primary carrier, and therefore his claim is submitted to that carrier. When Mrs. Smith goes to the dentist, Canada Life becomes the primary carrier; therefore, her claim is submitted to that company.

The patient copayment, if any, can then be claimed from the secondary carrier. If Mr. Smith's treatment amounts to $100 and he is required to pay $20 which is not reimbursable under his plan, he can then submit that $20 claim to Mrs. Smith's company for payment. What is required on the submission to the second carrier is a copy of the insurance claim form, clearly marked "duplicate," along with the "Explanation of Benefits" section attached to the cheque received from the primary carrier. This will provide the secondary carrier with proof that the primary carrier has been first to pay.

When there are dependent eligible members (e.g., children), the primary carrier is determined by the subscriber whose birthday is earliest in the calendar year. For example, if Mr. Smith was born on December 2 and Mrs. Smith was born on September 12, then Mrs. Smith's company becomes the primary carrier for the Smith children.

UNDERSTANDING THE FEE GUIDE

For each province there is a suggested fee guide listing various categories of services. These are intended only as suggested fees, not as a schedule. Dentists are not restricted as to what fees they can charge.

The fee guides contain the recommended fees that were established by dentists. A survey of dental procedures is taken each year and the time required for each is analyzed and averaged to arrive at what is considered to be a reasonable professional hourly fee. As a result of this information analysis, the fee guide provides dentists with charges that are considered to be **reasonable and customary** fees according to their relative value unit. In other words, a relative value has been assigned to the professional treatment time.

Services are identified through procedure codes that indicate to the insurance carrier what procedure was performed and what the usual fee is. Some procedures may be identified with IC beside the service description. This means that a relative value unit has not been identified; therefore, the procedure is subject to independent consideration. The dental office administrator is required to list the procedure codes on the dental insurance form and also identify the teeth and tooth surfaces involved. The dentist may provide the codes, or they may have to be looked up in the fee guide. A dental computer software program will contain the current year's fee guide and is quickly accessible to the administrator.

Although fees may vary from province to province, the categories of services are consistent in each province, and as demonstrated on the procedure codes listed in Table 7.1.

It is impossible to learn about every type of claim form that you may encounter. However, the Canadian Dental Association has standardized a format that is acceptable at all insurance companies. Individual claim forms may be provided by the insurance carrier, but in most cases the Standard Dental Claim Form is accepted.

Instructions for Completing Claim Forms

A. *Patient Information.* The dental office must fill out this section to identify the person for whom the services were rendered.

B. *Dentist Information.* This portion of the claim form may be pre-printed. The first line of this section will contain the dentist's name and professional degrees. If applicable, the dental group name will be printed on the next line. This will be followed by the dental office address. The final line will contain the dental office telephone number.

This section will also contain the unique number of each dentist. The Canadian Dental Association has approved a numbering system to identify each dentist, consisting of a six-digit number, which may be followed by a two-digit specialty code.

TABLE 7.1 **DENTAL PROCEDURE CODES**

PROCEDURE CODE	TYPE OF SERVICE
00000–09999	*Diagnostic*—includes radiographs, diagnostic study models, panoramic x-rays, bitewings, periapicals, etc.
10000–19999	*Preventive*—recall appointments, prophylaxis, pit and fissure sealants, etc.
20000–29999	*Restorative*—fillings, crowns, etc.
30000–39999	*Endodontics*—root canal therapy and associated treatment
40000–49999	*Periodontics*—scaling, root planing, surgical procedures, etc.
50000–59999	*Prosthodontics, Removable*—full and partial dentures, relines, etc.
60000–69999	*Prosthodontics, Fixed*—bridges, pontics, etc.
70000–79999	*Exodontics, Oral Surgery*—extractions, complicated and uncomplicated surgery
80000—89999	*Orthodontics*—orthodontic bands, braces, fixed and removable appliances
90000–99999	*Adjunctive General*—anaesthetic, general and conscious sedation

C. *Assignment of Benefits*. This clause should be signed only if the subscriber wishes to assign the benefit to the dentist. The patient must clearly understand that he or she is assigning payment to the dentist. In most provinces, assignment of benefits is discouraged by local dental associations.

D. *For Dentist's Use Only.* This section is used for additional information regarding diagnosis, procedures, or special considerations to explain the services listed on the claim form. Use this section freely if there is any doubt about the clarity of claim entries.

   The duplicate form should be checked if a second claim form is completed, for example, for coordination of benefits or in the event of a lost form.

E. *Patient Signature*. This section serves a dual purpose: When the patient (or parent/guardian) signs here, he or she authorizes release of information and acknowledges responsibility for the account. The release of information will allow the dentist to forward pertinent data via letters or radiographs when requested by a dental

EXHIBIT 7.2 STANDARD DENTAL CLAIM FORM

Canadian Dental Association

STANDARD DENTAL CLAIM FORM

Canadian Life and Health Insurance Association

PART 1 DENTIST

UNIQUE NO.	SPEC.	PATIENT'S OFFICE ACCOUNT NO.
345678		00044

I HEREBY ASSIGN MY BENEFITS PAYABLE FROM THIS CLAIM TO THE NAMED DENTIST AND AUTHORIZE PAYMENT DIRECTLY TO HIM/HER.

PATIENT
LAST NAME: *Patient, Mrs. Denise* GIVEN NAME
ADDRESS: *12 Scarth Street* APT.
CITY: *Hamilton, Ont.* PROV. POSTAL CODE: *L9L 9L9*

DENTIST
Dr. M. Molar
123 Cuspid Rd.
Hamilton, Ontario
L9K 9K9
PHONE NO. *(905) 555-2211*

SIGNATURE OF SUBSCRIBER

FOR DENTIST'S USE ONLY, FOR ADDITIONAL INFORMATION, DIAGNOSIS, PROCEDURES, OR SPECIAL CONSIDERATION.

I UNDERSTAND THAT THE FEES LISTED IN THIS CLAIM MAY NOT BE COVERED BY OR MAY EXCEED MY PLAN BENEFITS. I UNDERSTAND THAT I AM FINANCIALLY RESPONSIBLE TO MY DENTIST FOR THE ENTIRE TREATMENT.
I ACKNOWLEDGE THAT THE TOTAL FEE OF $ ____ IS ACCURATE AND HAS BEEN CHARGED TO ME FOR SERVICES RENDERED. I AUTHORIZE RELEASE OF THE INFORMATION CONTAINED IN THIS CLAIM FORM TO MY INSURING COMPANY/PLAN ADMINISTRATOR.

SIGNATURE OF PATIENT (PARENT GUARDIAN)

OFFICE VERIFICATION / DENTIST'S SIGNATURE *Dr. M. Molar, B.Sc., D.D.S.*

DUPLICATE FORM ☐

DATE OF SERVICE			PROCEDURE CODE	INTL. TOOTH CODE	TOOTH SURFACES	DENTIST'S FEE		LABORATORY CHARGE	TOTAL CHARGES	
DAY	MO.	YR.								
04	11	96	01103			87	06		87	06
04	11	96	21223	26	MOD	90	83		90	83

THIS IS AN ACCURATE STATEMENT OF SERVICES PERFORMED AND THE TOTAL FEE DUE AND PAYABLE. E.& OE.

TOTAL FEE SUBMITTED $177.89

INSTRUCTIONS
1. EMPLOYEE COMPLETE PARTS 2 AND 3.
2. HAVE YOUR DENTIST COMPLETE PART 1.
3. IF YOU WISH BENEFITS TO BE PAID DIRECTLY TO THE DENTIST, SIGN THE ASSIGNMENT PORTION OF PART 1 ABOVE. ASSIGNMENT OF BENEFITS IS IRREVOCABLE.
4. SEND THIS CLAIM FORM TO:

   ONTARIO:
   The Great-West Life Assurance Co.
   Hamilton Benefit Payment Office
   8th Floor, One King Street West
   Hamilton, Ontario
   L8P 4X9

   QUEBEC AND ATLANTIC PROVINCES:
   The Great-West Life Assurance Co.
   Montreal Benefit Payment Office
   P.O. Box 400
   Place Bonaventure
   Montreal, Quebec
   H5A 1B9

   WESTERN PROVINCES:
   The Great-West Life Assurance Co.
   Alberta Benefit Payment Office
   Suite 801
   10104-103 Ave.
   Edmonton, Alberta
   T5J 4R5

PART 2 EMPLOYEE INFORMATION

PLAN NO. *54180*   H.R. ID *12345-00*

NAME OF EMPLOYER OR GROUP *I. M. Ployer*

YOUR NAME: (PLEASE PRINT) *Denise* (FIRST) *Patient* (LAST)

YOUR DATE OF BIRTH: *01 / 01 / 62* DAY MONTH YEAR

I AUTHORIZE RELEASE OF ANY INFORMATION OR RECORD REQUESTED IN RESPECT OF THIS CLAIM TO GREAT-WEST LIFE OR ITS AGENTS AND CERTIFY THAT THE INFORMATION GIVEN IS TRUE, CORRECT AND COMPLETE TO THE BEST OF MY KNOWLEDGE.

EMPLOYEE'S SIGNATURE _____   DATE *Nov 4/96*

PART 3 PATIENT INFORMATION

1. PATIENT'S RELATIONSHIP TO YOU *same*   2. PATIENT'S DATE OF BIRTH *01 / 01 / 62* DAY MONTH YEAR
3. IF THE PATIENT IS A CHILD, DOES THE PATIENT RESIDE WITH YOU? YES ☐ NO ☐
4. IF THE PATIENT IS A CHILD OVER 19:

   IS HE/SHE A FULL-TIME STUDENT? YES ☐ NO ☐ IF YES, NAME OF SCHOOL _____
5. A) ARE YOU OR YOUR SPOUSE OR CHILD ENTITLED TO BENEFITS FROM ANY OTHER SOURCE? YES ☐ NO ☒

   IF YES, GIVE NAME AND ADDRESS OF OTHER SOURCE _____

   NAME OF FAMILY MEMBER INSURED _____ POLICY # _____

   B) IF YES TO A) ABOVE, AND THE PATIENT IS A DEPENDENT CHILD, PLEASE PROVIDE SPOUSE'S DATE OF BIRTH _____ DAY MONTH
6. IS TREATMENT REQUIRED AS THE RESULT OF AN ACCIDENT? YES ☐ NO ☒ IF YES, GIVE DATE, LOCATION, AND EXPLAIN HOW ACCIDENT HAPPENED _____
7. IF CLAIM IS FOR DENTURE, CROWN OR BRIDGE, IS THIS INITIAL PLACEMENT? YES ☐ NO ☒ IF NO, GIVE DATE OF PRIOR PLACEMENT AND REASON FOR REPLACEMENT _____

M445D(51160)-4/95   DC0726/726A

Sample provided by ABEL Computers Ltd., Burlington, Ontario.

consultant, without contravening any confidentiality of medical record laws. There is also a place here to enter the total amount of the account for which the patient acknowledges responsibility. This amount must equal the total fee submitted.

F. *Office Verification.* This section must be signed by the dentist or stamped with an official provincial dental association stamp. This verifies that the services itemized were performed.

G. *Services,* This section itemizes each service, the date of the treatment, tooth number, tooth surfaces, and dentist's fee.

H. *Laboratory Charge.* The Health Disciplines Act requires that the commercial laboratory charge must be separated from the dentist's professional fee. Each must be entered in their respective columns. Because many offices now have laboratories as part of their premises, the laboratory charge column is used only when an outside laboratory is involved. A commercial laboratory charge should never be rounded off to the nearest dollar. The patient should be charged the exact amount and the claim submitted accordingly. Only charges substantiated by a proper invoice from the dental laboratory should be charged under this column. It is advisable to block out all remaining unused lines of the procedure code column and the total charge column with an X to prevent any improper additions. Enter the sum of all professional and commercial laboratory fees beside the *Total Fee Submitted*.

Once the patient has signed the claim form, it becomes a statement of proof of services that have been performed. Although the dentist's signature is not a requirement for payment, the dentist is responsible for the accuracy of all information contained on the form.

The date of services on the dental claim form must be the exact date of the completion of the services. Changing this date is illegal; it must match the date recorded on the patient's chart when the service was completed.

ELECTRONIC DATA INTERCHANGE

Electronic Data Interchange (EDI) is the electronic submission of insurance claims. A dental office equipped to do so uses a computer program to transmit claim information electronically. Many dental offices find it quick and convenient to submit claims to those insurance carriers that will accept EDI.

When a claim is sent electronically, the insurance carrier acknowledges receipt of the claim and responds, via modem, giving the status of the claim. When the claim has been accepted and acknowledged, the patient can expect to receive payment sooner, sometimes within a few days. If the practice accepts assigned claims, then payment will be directed to the dental office.

The advantages of EDI claim submissions are that they speed up claim processing, allow prompt error correction, provide immediate claims calculations, and reduce paperwork. To find out which insurance carriers accept EDI submissions, the dental office administrator can contact the Canadian Dental Association.

ASSIGNMENT

1. What does it mean if an office does not accept assignment?
2. In the provincial fee guide, under what category would you find the following procedures:
   a. full mouth x-rays _____
   b. six-month recall (adult) _____
   c. three-surface amalgam _____
   d. an extraction _____
   e. a crown _____
3. When should a predetermination form be completed? _____
   _____
4. Complete a Standard Dental Claim form (p. 85) with the following information:

Patient:	Molly Molar	Doctor:	Dr. D. Kay
	123 Cuspid Court		155 Caries Street
	Your city, Province		Your city, Province
	L9N 1K9		L3N 2K9
			Phone no. 555-1212
			I.D. # 123334

Molly attended Dr. Kay's office on March 29/96 and had the following services performed:

Initial exam—01203 permanent dentition

Full mouth series radiographs—02112

Prophylaxis,2 TU (time units)—11300

Amalgam filling on tooth no. 4.4, DO—21222

Amalgam filling on tooth no. 2.7, MOD—21223

5. Describe how the dental office administrator can assist the patient with understanding his or her insurance benefit and what is meant by informed choice.

6. When a patient calls for a recall/hygiene appointment, what should the dental office administrator check before scheduling the appointment?

STANDARD DENTAL CLAIM FORM

Canadian Dental Association

STANDARD DENTAL CLAIM FORM

Canadian Life and Health Insurance Association

PART 1 DENTIST

| UNIQUE NO. | SPEC. | PATIENT'S OFFICE ACCOUNT NO. |

I HEREBY ASSIGN MY BENEFITS PAYABLE FROM THIS CLAIM TO THE NAMED DENTIST AND AUTHORIZE PAYMENT DIRECTLY TO HIM/HER.

PATIENT

LAST NAME   GIVEN NAME

ADDRESS   APT.

CITY   PROV.   POSTAL CODE

DENTIST

PHONE NO.

SIGNATURE OF SUBSCRIBER

FOR DENTIST'S USE ONLY, FOR ADDITIONAL INFORMATION, DIAGNOSIS, PROCEDURES, OR SPECIAL CONSIDERATION.

I UNDERSTAND THAT THE FEES LISTED IN THIS CLAIM MAY NOT BE COVERED BY OR MAY EXCEED MY PLAN BENEFITS. I UNDERSTAND THAT I AM FINANCIALLY RESPONSIBLE TO MY DENTIST FOR THE ENTIRE TREATMENT.
I ACKNOWLEDGE THAT THE TOTAL FEE OF $ _____ IS ACCURATE AND HAS BEEN CHARGED TO ME FOR SERVICES RENDERED. I AUTHORIZE RELEASE OF THE INFORMATION CONTAINED IN THIS CLAIM FORM TO MY INSURING COMPANY/PLAN ADMINISTRATOR.

SIGNATURE OF PATIENT (PARENT GUARDIAN)

OFFICE VERIFICATION / DENTIST'S SIGNATURE

DUPLICATE FORM ☐

DATE OF SERVICE			PROCEDURE CODE	INTL. TOOTH CODE	TOOTH SURFACES	DENTIST'S FEE	LABORATORY CHARGE	TOTAL CHARGES
DAY	MO.	YR.						

THIS IS AN ACCURATE STATEMENT OF SERVICES PERFORMED AND THE TOTAL FEE DUE AND PAYABLE, E.& O.E.

TOTAL FEE SUBMITTED

INSTRUCTIONS

1. EMPLOYEE COMPLETE PARTS 2 AND 3.
2. HAVE YOUR DENTIST COMPLETE PART 1.
3. IF YOU WISH BENEFITS TO BE PAID DIRECTLY TO THE DENTIST, SIGN THE ASSIGNMENT PORTION OF PART 1 ABOVE. ASSIGNMENT OF BENEFITS IS IRREVOCABLE.
4. SEND THIS CLAIM FORM TO:

ONTARIO:
The Great-West Life Assurance Co.
Hamilton Benefit Payment Office
8th Floor, One King Street West
Hamilton, Ontario
L8P 4X9

QUEBEC AND ATLANTIC PROVINCES:
The Great-West Life Assurance Co.
Montreal Benefit Payment Office
P.O. Box 400
Place Bonaventure
Montreal, Quebec
H5A 1B9

WESTERN PROVINCES:
The Great-West Life Assurance Co.
Alberta Benefit Payment Office
Suite 801
10104-103 Ave.
Edmonton, Alberta
T5J 4R5

PART 2 EMPLOYEE INFORMATION

PLAN NO. _____   H.R. ID _____

NAME OF EMPLOYER OR GROUP _____

YOUR NAME: (PLEASE PRINT) _____ (FIRST) _____ (LAST)

YOUR DATE OF BIRTH: ___ / ___ / ___   DAY   MONTH   YEAR

I AUTHORIZE RELEASE OF ANY INFORMATION OR RECORD REQUESTED IN RESPECT OF THIS CLAIM TO GREAT-WEST LIFE OR ITS AGENTS AND CERTIFY THAT THE INFORMATION GIVEN IS TRUE, CORRECT AND COMPLETE TO THE BEST OF MY KNOWLEDGE.

EMPLOYEE'S SIGNATURE _____   DATE _____

PART 3 PATIENT INFORMATION

1. PATIENT'S RELATIONSHIP TO YOU _____   2. PATIENT'S DATE OF BIRTH ___ / ___ / ___   DAY   MONTH   YEAR

3. IF THE PATIENT IS A CHILD, DOES THE PATIENT RESIDE WITH YOU?   YES ☐   NO ☐

4. IF THE PATIENT IS A CHILD OVER 19:

   IS HE/SHE A FULL-TIME STUDENT?   YES ☐   NO ☐   IF YES, NAME OF SCHOOL _____

5. A) ARE YOU OR YOUR SPOUSE OR CHILD ENTITLED TO BENEFITS FROM ANY OTHER SOURCE?   YES ☐   NO ☐

   IF YES, GIVE NAME AND ADDRESS OF OTHER SOURCE

   _____

   NAME OF FAMILY MEMBER INSURED _____   POLICY # _____

   B) IF YES TO A) ABOVE, AND THE PATIENT IS A DEPENDENT CHILD, PLEASE PROVIDE SPOUSE'S DATE OF BIRTH _____   DAY   MONTH

6. IS TREATMENT REQUIRED AS THE RESULT OF AN ACCIDENT?   YES ☐   NO ☐   IF YES, GIVE DATE, LOCATION, AND EXPLAIN HOW ACCIDENT HAPPENED _____

7. IF CLAIM IS FOR DENTURE, CROWN OR BRIDGE, IS THIS INITIAL PLACEMENT?   YES ☐   NO ☐   IF NO, GIVE DATE OF PRIOR PLACEMENT AND REASON FOR REPLACEMENT _____

M445D(51160)-4/95   DC0726/726A

Sample provided by ABEL Computers Ltd., Burlington, Ontario.

CHAPTER EIGHT

APPOINTMENT SCHEDULING

OBJECTIVE

At the end of this chapter, the student will be able to identify and describe the following: how to create an ideal day, schedule appointments for the dentist and hygienist, and double book using a two-operatory system; how to handle changes in the schedule and identify and acknowledge the needs of the patient and the dentist.

TOPICS

- scheduling time units/buffer zones
- creating a matrix
- goal setting, creating the ideal day
- double booking
- managing the stress level, maintaining patient flow
- cancellation list/short notice list
- confirming appointments
- scheduling hygiene appointments
- managing dental emergencies

KEY TO PRODUCTIVITY

Appointment scheduling is the responsibility of the administrative staff and is one of the most important and challenging activities. It takes dedication, commitment, and skill. The skill involves knowing where every member of the office is and what each is doing. In addition, the administrator needs to know where the patients are and what administrative support they need. A finely tuned dental team will work together in synchronized harmony to provide high quality care for a well-balanced flow of patients, while keeping the office stress level to a minimum.

The dentist and staff should begin with a complete analysis of the dental practice to determine the potential for financial productivity according to the office philosophy regarding the delivery of dental care. The staff should set goals that will maximize production, minimize stress, and meet the needs of the patient in a unified effort. A well-organized dental office administrator will be a key player in this process.

THE APPOINTMENT BOOK

A manual appointment book is sometimes used in dental offices, whether or not there is a computerized system. It is still one of the most efficient and effective methods of scheduling. Although many dental software companies have developed very good appointment schedulers with built in ticklers or reminder systems, it is essential for the dental office administrator to understand all aspects of manual appointment scheduling in order to make good use of electronic media.

Selecting an Appointment Book

A few features that you would consider when selecting an appointment book are as follows:

1. It should contain an appropriate number of columns based on the number of operatories or treatment rooms available.
2. It should be set up with appropriate time units. A time unit (TU) is an increment of the day, usually 10 or 15 minutes. The most common time unit is 10 minutes.
3. The appointment book contains confidential information; therefore, security should be considered to protect it.
4. The size and design of the appointment book will be determined by the amount of counter or desk space that is available.
5. An appointment book designed to show a "week at a glance" allows the administrator to quickly note openings in the week.
6. The appointment book should provide enough pages for a full year so that holidays and vacations can be blocked off in advance.

7. There should be sufficient space within each column to print the necessary information for each patient, including the telephone number.

8. Colour coded pages are helpful for instant identification of days of the week.

Factors to Consider

Office Hours and Lunch Hours

Diagonal lines should be made across the hours that the office is not open, as well as the lunch hour, when creating the matrix (advance schedule). Occasionally a clinical staff member will schedule an appointment for a patient and it is easy to schedule incorrectly if the hours of operation are not clearly defined.

The dentist and staff should decide on the best time for the lunch hour and if the office should remain open during this period. Most offices will stagger the lunch hours so that someone will be at the front desk at all times, but all dental staff get a break.

Many dental practices have extended hours of operation to accommodate patients who are working during normal business hours. This will mean that the working hours of the employees will be staggered.

SCHEDULING APPOINTMENTS

All appointments should be scheduled in pencil, never in ink. There will be numerous changes to the schedule during the day and pencil is much easier to erase. All appointment book entries should be accurate, legible, and complete. They should include all information necessary for the clinical staff to prepare for the appointment. It is ideal if one person is responsible for all entries made in the appointment book.

Here are some guidelines for appointment scheduling:

1. Print appointment entries in pencil. Everyone has different handwriting and it is time-consuming to try to decipher it. This wastes valuable time.

2. Print the patient's last name first. This will be helpful when pulling charts.

3. Include the patient's home and/or business telephone number for confirmation calls.

4. Indicate whether the patient is an adult or a child. For example, Mr., Mrs., or Ms. would indicate an adult and no title would indicate a child. Messages should not be left with children.
5. Note the treatment being done on the schedule so that clinical staff can prepare for it.
6. Verify that laboratory work has been received before the patient is in the chair.
7. Note whether the patient is to be premedicated or has a medical condition that would affect treatment.
8. Indicate the length of the appointment with a vertical line or arrow.
9. Identify new patients. You should ask the new patient to come in a few minutes early to complete a medical history form and at that time should welcome him or her to the practice (refer to p. 93 for information on new patient procedure).

Confirming Appointments

All appointments should be confirmed the previous day. As a courtesy to the patient, when an appointment is made, ask if he or she would like to be called to confirm it. Some patients may be offended at receiving reminder calls. If so, indicate preconfirmation on the schedule with a check mark. Always repeat the appointment date and time orally to the patient along with written confirmation in the form of an appointment card.

All other patients should be called the day before to confirm their appointments. This process reduces the number of patients who do not show up because they forgot. If an appointment time has unexpectedly become inconvenient for a patient, then there is sufficient time to schedule another (perhaps using the short notice list).

EXHIBIT 8.1 **SAMPLE APPOINTMENT BOOK ENTRY**

8:00	Doe, John
8:15	Aml. 2.6
8:30	555-1212
8:45	Jones, Mabel
9:00	N/P exam
9:15	3 TU, 555-3333

EXHIBIT 8.2 APPOINTMENT PHONE LIST

Printed 03/MAR/95 02.26p
Accounting Date: 03/MAR/95

Family Dental Centre
From: 03/MAR/95   To: 03/MAR/95

Patient	Phone No.s	PID	Age	Appt. with	Reason	Chair	Time	Units	Date
Mr. Jerry Chapman 44 Worthington Way Burlington, Ontario L4K 5C3	(905)634–1348 >(905)434–3330	10502	65	John Hollis, B.A., D.D.S. chk **MEDICAL WARNING-SEE CHART** pen. allergy		1	08:00a	1	03/MAR/95
Leslie Anderson R.,R. #2 Caledonia, Ontario L0H 1G0	(905)234–2528 >(905)643–3386	08634	26	John Hollis, B.A., D.D.S. rest likes nitrous		1	08:30a	3	03/MAR/95
Mrs. Kathy Plonyski 718 Chatsworth Place Burlington, Ontario L7P 2E2	(905)389–7364 >(905)343–7544 noon	06885	74	John Hollis, B.A., D.D.S. lost rest **MEDICAL WARNING-SEE CHART** Penicillin allergy		1	09:00a	3	03/MAR/95
Miss Vanna M. Montreal 119 Jean Worrel Cres Hamilton, Ontario L7K 6T5	>(905)332–3000 (905)246–4233	08415	32	John Hollis, B.A., D.D.S. 3 needs rest Waitress		1	10:00a	3	03/MAR/95
Mr. John Sandelli 969 Warburton Burlington, Ontario L7M 8L1	(905)547–7848 >(905)542–3013 lunch	10109	36	John Hollis, B.A.,D.D.S. rest was 28FEB95 hates dentists		1	10:30a	6	03/MAR/95
Mr. Johnny A. Walker 235 Main St. E. Hamilton, Ontario L0H 1T0	>(905)375–6731 (905)547–5461 after 5	03224	58	John Hollis, B.A.,D.D.S. lost rest referred by Joe F.		1	11:30a	3	03/MAR/95
Mr. Joel Pitcher 629 Forest Hill (905)234–2100 L7M 7N6	>(905)384–1944	02442	44	John Hollis, B.A.,D.D.S. crown prep ins pay 50% ask for payment up front!		1	01:00p	21	03/MAR/95 Toronto, Ontario
Mr. Scott E. Goodyear Box 78 Burlington, Ontario L0K 3N0	>(905)377–6475 (905)342–3581 9am	01162	47	John Hollis, B.A.,D.D.S. prob with gum abcess?! **MEDICAL WARNING-SEE CHART** scared		1	04:30p	2	03/MAR/95
Mrs. Mary M. Suess 3310 South Service Road Burlington, Ontario L7M 3K5	>(905)555–1212	02993	67	Sharon Giles, R.D.H. rc/B*L		3	09:00a	4	03/MAR/95

Sample provided by ABEL Computers Ltd., Burlington, Ontario.

PREPARING FOR APPOINTMENTS

Once appointments are scheduled, the following preparations can be made the day before:

1. Confirm appointments and indicate confirmation on the schedule with a check mark.
2. Pull the charts at least one day ahead.
3. Check all charts for medical alerts.
4. Check account balances for outstanding amounts.
5. Check to see if there are predeterminations outstanding.
6. Check to see if medical histories should be updated.
7. Check to see if special insurance forms are needed and if patient is near the annual maximum.
8. File the charts in chronological order (according to the time the patients are coming in) and lock the charts in a fireproof cabinet.
9. Photocopy a schedule for each treatment room, each "make ready" area, and the dentist's office. A "make ready" area is usually between the treatment rooms where instrument trays are prepared and instruments are sterilized.
10. Colour code the schedules.

Colour Coding Schedules

Colour coding the photocopied schedules and posting them in every treatment area is a valuable time-saving procedure. To begin, select three coloured highlighters. Each colour will be used to identify chart locations. For example:

Green—indicates a new patient

Yellow —indicates that the patient is seeing the dentist and the hygienist

Pink—indicates a medical condition/alert

Colour coding will assist the clinical staff in knowing where the charts are. A new patient, for example, will not have a chart prepared. The green notation will help to remind the office administrator to begin preparing the new patient's chart and to allow time for the new patient procedure.

The appointment that is highlighted in yellow will remind the dental assistant not to release the patient until he or she sees the hygienist.

In this case, the chart should be moved into the hygienist's treatment room, and the patient may be asked to wait in the reception area. The pink (or red) highlighter will indicate that a patient has a medical condition which the dentist should be alerted to. If the patient requires prophylactic antibiotics, for example, then the dentist can verify that the medication presents no danger before commencing treatment.

The colours may vary, but it is important to use them consistently. All of the clinical staff should know the meaning of the colour codes. The clinical staff can then see at a glance the structure of the day and determine the location of the charts.

CANCELLATION AND SHORT NOTICE LISTS

Occasionally a patient may need to cancel an appointment. When patients are familiar with the office policy regarding cancellations, very few will cancel or not show up for appointments. Appointments should always be made at a time that is convenient for the patient and the service provider. However, patients should be asked to provide the office with 24–48 hours notice if they need to cancel. That will allow the office administrator time to call another patient to fill the appointment time.

A "short notice" list should be kept at the front of the appointment book. This is a list of patients who can be called, and would like to be called, at short notice. Ask each patient if he or she would like to be placed on the short notice list in the event that a preferred time should become available. When a patient is called from the short notice list, try to avoid using the word "cancellation." That indicates that it is acceptable to cancel appointments. More appropriate wording would be "change of schedule." For example, "Mrs. Smith, the doctor has had a change in schedule today and I immediately thought of you. I know that you like morning appointments and this is ideally suited for you." This leaves the patient with the impression that the dental office administrator is going out of his or her way to accommodate the patient.

If a patient simply does not show up for a scheduled appointment, every effort should be made to contact that person. Remind him or her of the office policy regarding missed appointments. The patient's name should go on a cancellation list. If no attempt is made to contact these patients, they may feel that their treatment is not necessary or may not understand the value of keeping scheduled appointments.

EXHIBIT 8.3 MISSED APPOINTMENTS

MISSED APPOINTMENTS

Printed: 03?MAR/95 04:31p
Accounting Date: 03/MAR/95

From: 03/MAR/95   To: 03/MAR/95

Date	Col	Time	Pvdr	Work-to-do	Patient	
03/MAR/95	1	07:10p	H	rest13,44	BELL, Mrs. Wendy, 176 New St.	H (905)342–9546
03/MAR/95	1	07:50p	H	rest	BURGMAN, Mrs. Lee E., 767–5454 Sheppard Ave.	H (416)653–6300
03/MAR/95	3	07:40p	S	rc/c*h	POIRIER, Jack, 4357 Leslie St.	W (905) 342–3230
03/MAR/95	3	08:20p	S	rc B*H	HASLAM, MR. JOE, 64 Regent Street	W (905)535–3300
03/MAR/95	B	07:30p	Z	rc/a*h	JONES, Katie E., Box 9	H (905)343–2085
03/MAR/95	B	08:00p	Z	rc/a*h	SMITH, Emelia J., 3232 Bond St.	H (905)433–2065

Sample provided by ABEL Computers Ltd., Burlington, Ontario.

NEW PATIENT PROCEDURE

New patients should be asked to arrive at the dental office 5 to 10 minutes in advance of their appointment. They are required to complete forms providing the administrator with demographic and insurance information and a complete medical history. New patients can be given a brochure outlining the policies and philosophy of the dental office.

The new patient procedure is vital to the success of a dental office as it will convey the tone, image, and philosophy for the office. It will allow the office administrator to establish good office policies in advance as well as to provide good patient service. This is an opportunity to discuss the patient's dental insurance program, provide assistance, and educate the patient on the practice policies such as the confirmation of appointments, new patient exam, ongoing care, hygiene appointments, and missed appointments. The information provided to the dentist will be helpful in structuring the treatment time to provide maximum care and benefit to the patient. The new patient experience is crucial to the overall success of the future relationship.

DETERMINE AND PLAN THE IDEAL DAY

Communication with the dental care providers is absolutely essential to the success of effective appointment scheduling. You should ask the dentist and hygienists how they like their day to be set up—in other words, what is their "ideal" day. The ideal day should be compatible with the preset productivity goals. It is often difficult to achieve an ideal day because of interruptions or emergencies. However, it does provide a starting point and a guideline to follow when looking at the day in its entirety.

The clinical staff can provide estimates of the usual time required for specific procedures. The hygiene staff should inform the administrative staff how long they require for an adult recall appointment, pit and fissure sealants, children's recall appointments, etc.

It is most important for the dental office administrator to remember not to book too many difficult appointments close together. Doing so will cause the service provider to "burn out." If the dentist has just completed an extensive surgical procedure, then the next appointment should be something "light," such as an examination or minor procedure of some kind. Treatment rooms may need to be set up and dental instruments changed and sterilized between appointments.

Ask the dentist when he or she prefers to do specific procedures. For example, some may prefer to perform more complicated procedures in the morning, when they are rested, and reserve the afternoon for lighter appointments such as new patient examinations or fillings.

When scheduling appointments with patients, take the opportunity to educate them and reinforce treatment times while maintaining control of the schedule. For example, "we like to do that procedure between 10:00 a.m. and noon and the next opening we have is ...."

Try to create an ideal day and customize it to the needs of the patient as well as the doctor. Remember to allow time for sterilization of instruments and for the clinical staff to "catch their breath." If the day is scheduled to maximum capacity, make arrangements to assist with setting up instrument trays, cleanup, sterilization, or whatever is needed. Clinical staff are generally very willing to demonstrate how to set up instrument trays and operate sterilization equipment. Your assistance will help to alleviate the stress which accompanies busy and highly productive days and reinforce the team concept to all staff members.

Set Goals for Financial Productivity

The dental office administrator should always be aware of how much productivity is necessary to keep the practice viable. It is helpful for the administrator to set financial goals. When a patient cancels an appointment or if there are spaces in the day's schedule, then downtime occurs.

Effective appointment scheduling can eliminate unproductive downtime and increase the financial productivity of a practice.

When downtime does occur due to unforeseen circumstances, the staff and/or the dentist can use this time for administration tasks, such as calling in prescriptions, planning treatment, or perhaps following up on predeterminations.

Double Booking

If a dentist has two dental assistants and works in two operatories or treatment rooms, downtime will be greatly reduced. As one patient's treatment is being completed, another patient is being seated and prepared for treatment. This system will allow the dentist to be "double booked." This system should be used with extreme caution. Remember that neither the dentist nor the patient can be in two places at the same time.

For example, in Operatory 1, the first five minutes of the first time unit is spent with the dental assistant seating the patient, placing the x-rays on the x-ray viewer, and putting the bib on the patient, along with general conversation. At this time the dentist is not needed in the treatment room. The dentist then enters the treatment room and administers anaesthetic or begins the procedure. Assume that when dentist time is indicated, the dentist cannot leave the treatment area where the patient is.

While the dentist works in one room, a patient should not be scheduled in the second treatment room unless only the assistant is needed. Understanding this takes practice and the ability to visualize where everyone is. A great deal of thought is required for every appointment that is scheduled in a double booking system.

Emergency versus Urgency

It is difficult to determine over the telephone if a dental "emergency" is a true emergency or simply an urgency. An emergency should be attended to immediately, whereas an urgency should be attended to as soon as possible, today or perhaps tomorrow. For example, an emergency would be an abscessed tooth causing a fever and swelling, whereas an urgency would be a pre-existing condition which may be chronic rather than acute.

There are specific questions that can help to differentiate between an emergency and an urgency. Refer to Chapter 9 for some examples.

EXHIBIT 8.4 **SAMPLE APPOINTMENT SCHEDULE**

"O" indicates assistant time "X" indicates dentist time			
OPERATORY 1		**OPERATORY 2**	
9:00 a.m. Doe, Jane	O X		
9:15 a.m. Root canal therapy ✓	X		
9:30 a.m. 4 TU	X		
9:45 a.m. (Home phone) 555-1213	X O	Brown, George	O X
10:00 a.m.		3 TU, AML, 555-3434 ✓	X
10:15 a.m. Smith, Susan ✓		business 555-4554	O
10:30 a.m. Emerg. (Pain URQ)			

If the situation is an emergency, the patient should be told to come in right away or during the emergency buffer period. If the dentist is not available, the patient should be directed to a local hospital emergency department.

Buffer Zones

Buffer zones are usually reserved for emergencies. A buffer zone normally consists of one or two time units scheduled either in the morning or the afternoon, often just before or after lunch. If this time is not used for an emergency, it allows the dentist to catch up, if necessary, or it can be used for treatment planning. When a dental emergency does occur, schedule the patient in this time unit first. This time should not be considered a break time for staff or extended lunch hour.

Staff Meetings

Time should be set aside regularly (depending on the office policy) for dental team meetings. These should be held when they will not interfere with patient care. From time to time, the dentist may request that they be held over a lunch hour, in which case the office must be closed. Most team meetings are held toward the end of the day.

SCHOOL HOLIDAYS

A calendar of holidays is available from the school boards in your area. Many parents would like you to schedule their children during holidays or after school so that the child will not be absent too frequently. This is particularly important when scheduling a series of appointments for a child, as in orthodontic treatment. If you know when all of the school holidays are, you can offer a time that will accommodate the patient as well as the practice.

School holiday periods can be highly productive for dental offices. It is preferable to have a full staff during these periods who are prepared to be busy. These production periods are a perfect opportunity for the well-organized dental office administrator to effectively schedule all of the dental providers for optimal productivity.

SERIES OF APPOINTMENTS

Scheduling a patient for a series of appointments should not be done too far in advance. Try to schedule the next appointment on the same day of the week and at the same time as the original one. This reduces the chance of the patient not showing up for the scheduled appointment.

SCHEDULING PATIENTS WITH SPECIAL NEEDS

Young children are usually at their best in the morning after they have received proper rest and are alert and happy. Remember that whenever you have a child by the hand, you have the adult by the heart. A patient's earliest experiences in the dental office will affect future treatment and cooperation; therefore, they should be positive.

A nervous patient is more likely to cooperate in the morning, because he or she is prevented from anticipating the appointment all day long. If allowed to, the nervous patient may cancel or not show up at all with the whole day to think of excuses.

Elderly patients are generally at their best later in the morning or mid-afternoon. Patients who suffer from rheumatoid arthritis will awaken with stiff and sore joints, and therefore require extra time in the morning.

Elderly patients may have special transportation needs as well. Many of these patients live alone and the trip to the dental office could be a main event in their day, so they may wish to talk. Schedule them in at a time where you may have an extra minute or two to speak with them. This small act of kindness will create a positive experience for your elderly patients.

TIME MANAGEMENT

If the dentist is running late, the office administrator should tell the patient that the dentist has been delayed and approximately how long the delay will be. Displaying respect for the patient's time encourages patients to respond favourably by respecting the dentist's time. Patients left to wait for an extended period may feel ignored or overlooked and may become angry and impatient. In most cases, patients who are acknowledged are willing to wait and will leave the office with the impression that they have been well cared for. If it is impossible for a patient to stay, offer to reschedule the appointment and apologize for the inconvenience.

Late Patients

An office policy should be established regarding patients who arrive late for their appointments. The dentist and staff should agree on what procedure to follow if the patient arrives 10 minutes late, 30 minutes late, or even an hour late.

It is recommended that if a patient who is usually prompt arrives a few minutes late, he or she should be seen. From time to time it may be necessary to remind patients about the importance of keeping scheduled appointments and arriving on time. Be polite and understanding as the patient could have been held up in traffic or there could be some other valid reason for tardiness.

If a patient is 30 minutes late or more, the appointment should be rescheduled. Politely explain that because he or she did not arrive at the scheduled time, it was necessary to begin treatment for another patient who had been waiting.

Continuing Care Appointments

Continuing care appointments affect the financial productivity of the practice. The implementation of an effective system can begin with the communications between the patient and the hygienist and should be continually reinforced by the entire dental team. The hygienist helps to reinforce the importance of continuing care to patients and encourages acceptance of prebooking. The hygienist can stress the importance of preventive health care and tell patients that he or she looks forward to seeing them again in six months. The hygienist's attitude will promote the patient's acceptance.

When the patient schedules an appointment six months in advance, point out that this is to ensure that you are reserving the patient's preferred time. While scheduling the appointment, ask the patient to complete a self-addressed postcard. File the postcard for the month of the appointment and mail cards one month in advance. When patients receive cards in their own handwriting, it attracts their attention and reconfirms the commitment that they made to the dental office to keep their appointments. This procedure can save the dental office staff a great deal of time on the telephone calling patients to remind them that they are due for continuing care appointments.

CHANGING FROM MANUAL TO COMPUTERIZED SCHEDULING

When changing from a manual to an electronic system of appointment scheduling, the office should maintain a manual system for a minimum of six months. The manual system will provide an excellent backup in the event of problems common to newly installed computer systems. Electronic schedulers can provide call lists and reminder systems that help to maintain excellent organization.

ASSIGNMENT

You are scheduling for Dr. D. Kay. Dr. Kay uses two operatories and two assistants. There is one hygienist, S. Kaler. Office hours are from 8:00 a.m. to 4:00 p.m., and lunch is from noon to 1:00 p.m. Buffer times are before and after lunch.

1. Set up a schedule with the following appointments.

   Patient 1 needs to come in for a crown and bridge appointment. The bridge is from tooth no. 24 to 26. He needs 6 TU (time units) with the dentist.

   Patient 2 needs an uncomplicated extraction of tooth no. 2.5—2 TU.

   Patient 3 needs an amalgam on tooth no. 16, MOD—2 TU.

Patient 4 needs tooth no. 4.8 extracted (it will be complicated).

Patient 5 needs a recall exam, scale/prophylaxis, and two bitewing x-rays.

Patient 6 calls, feels feverish, is experiencing severe discomfort, feels sensitivity to heat (use emergency time).

Patient 7 will be coming in for her regular orthodontic adjustment, needs 2 TU.

Patient 8 needs a first appointment for dentures.

Patient 9 requires endodontic therapy on tooth no. 3.5, needs 2 TU.

Patient 10 needs an amalgam filling on tooth no. 3.7, MO, needs 2 TU.

Patient 11 requires pit and fissure sealants, 2 TU with the hygienist and 1 TU with the dentist for a minor exam.

Patient 12 requires 3 TU for a continuing care appointment with the hygienist and 2 TU for an amalgam filling with the dentist.

Patient 13 is a new patient. He will require 2 TU with the dentist for a new patient examination and 3 TU with the hygienist for scaling and prophylaxis.

2. Colour code the appointment schedule using the suggested colours.

APPOINTMENT SCHEDULE

			DATE		
			8	00	
				15	
				30	
				45	
			9	00	
				15	
				30	
				45	
			10	00	
				15	
				30	
				45	
			11	00	
				15	
				30	
				45	
			12	00	
				15	
				30	
				45	
			1	00	
				15	
				30	
				45	
			2	00	
				15	
				30	
				45	
			3	00	
				15	
				30	
				45	
			4	00	
				15	
				30	
				45	
			5	00	
				15	
				30	
				45	

Reproduced with permission by Safeguard Business Systems, Inc., Fort Washington, PA 19034

CHAPTER NINE

EFFECTIVE TELEPHONE SKILLS

OBJECTIVE

At the end of this chapter, the student will be able to identify and describe the following: how to organize a telephone communication system, prepare for incoming and outgoing calls, create a professional image through telephone communications, and provide legal protection for the dental office through appropriate telephone triage.

TOPICS

- public relations
- voice quality
- anatomy of the telephone call
- organizing a telephone system
- handling the angry caller
- telephone triage
- dental emergency versus urgency
- time management
- equipment
- types of calls

FRONT LINE OF COMMUNICATIONS

The telephone represents the front line of communications in the dental office. Its use or misuse will affect the patient/office relationship, the quality of dental care, and the growth of the practice. Telephone communications represent 30 to 50 percent of the patient's experience with the dental office, and yet they are often overlooked as vital to the viability of the practice. It is essential that the right person is selected for this responsibility, someone willing to perfect the skill of verbal communication. Having the wrong person in this position can be disastrous.

The person on the telephone is the goodwill representative and public relations contact for the dental office. This person is the liaison between the clinical environment and the business environment who has only one opportunity to make the first impression a good one. Patients who call cannot judge the practice by visual impressions of the staff, the equipment, or the office. They can only rely on the words that they hear to form their opinions.

Face-to-face communication consists of many nonverbal gestures, such as facial expression, body language, and eye contact, that combine with words to form and clarify the complete message. Telephone communications are absent of gestures, so the words that are used and the way they are spoken become even more important. Telephone communications don't allow the caller to form an impression from body language. It is therefore more important to concentrate on vocal quality along with the words used during each telephone encounter. There is no time for second thoughts. The quality of the communication depends on the skill and preparation of the dental office staff.

All forms of communication, whether written or verbal, should be clear, concise, and complete. To perfect effective telephone communications, the dental office administrator must plan ahead for all forms of incoming and outgoing calls. Preparing written protocols and providing proper training will help prepare every dental team member to handle specific situations. This process also serves to protect the dental office from the legal risk of malpractice arising from improper use of the telephone and incorrect collection of clinically significant information.

Voice Quality

The quality of your voice should reflect the quality of your life. Voice quality is a reflection of your own complex personality, and its warmth and friendliness should provide comfort to the dental patient. Patients should feel that they are communicating with a calm and mature professional who exercises sound judgment and compassion.

The dental office administrator should emphasize and use positive language at all times and avoid improper grammar and slang. The proper pronunciation of words and an even rate of speed are important to correct interpretation of your message. You should always sound alert, interested, natural, and distinct.

Voice quality is enhanced with good posture, pleasant facial expression, and a positive mental attitude. Using hand gestures helps to make the tone more expressive. The dental office may incorporate a variety of teaching methods for the dental staff, such as role playing or critiquing tapes, to judge the effectiveness of the telephone communications. Some offices may provide an audio script, which should be practised until it becomes natural.

Telephone communications are an extension of clinical care and often become the focal point for patient dissatisfaction. The dental office administrator must be prepared for the stress of handling a large volume of incoming and outgoing calls.

To be an effective communicator, one must be a responsive listener. Responsive listening requires concentration and planning. Providing callers with feedback and paraphrasing when appropriate helps them feel that they are being understood. The dental office administrator should ask appropriate probing questions and listen to each response without interruption.

TABLE 9.1 **SAMPLE PHRASES**

DO SAY	AVOID SAYING
I will find out ...	I don't know ...
Here is what we can do ...	We can't do that ...
Yes ...	OK ...
Certainly ...	Yeah ...
May I have the correct spelling. ...	Can you spell that for me ...
We have had a change in schedule ...	There has been a cancellation ...
Where is the discomfort ... ?	Where is the pain ... ?
I have seen ... (or I saw)	I seen ...
I have done ... (or I did)	I done ...
May I put you on hold ... ?	Hold please! (click) ...

ANATOMY OF THE TELEPHONE CALL

Telephone communications require skill, experience, and concentration. Understanding the nature and purpose of each type of call helps the dental office administrator to plan accordingly.

The essential components of each telephone call, whether incoming or outgoing, are as follows:

1. Greeting
2. Gathering information
3. Closure

The greeting consists of an introduction to the office. It should include the name of the office and the name of the person to whom the caller is speaking. Most dental patients prefer to speak to an identified person rather than to a department. An offer of help should be included in the greeting. For example, "Good morning, Dr. Jones' office, Sally speaking. How may I help you?"

This greeting assures the caller that he or she has called the correct office and the administrator is prepared to help.

Gathering relevant information requires skill because accuracy is significant for the appropriate treatment of the patient. The dental office administrator must often make immediate decisions regarding the nature of the call. A well-informed administrator will ask appropriate questions to determine if the call is an emergency or an urgency. It is helpful to review with the dentist how specific situations should be handled. (See Emergency versus Urgency below.)

The third part of the telephone encounter is the closure. It is at this point that action is called for. An offer to help is made by making an appointment, taking a message, or referring the patient to another source. Once the action has been commenced, all efforts should be made to complete it. If the action requires follow-up later, then it should be taken care of.

EMERGENCY VERSUS URGENCY

When a patient is experiencing discomfort, it is an urgent matter. To determine the nature of the call requires sound judgment and calmness. You must decide if the patient needs to see the dentist immediately (an emergency) or if the patient can be scheduled in during a buffer zone or at the first available opening (an urgency). The most important information to be gathered immediately is the name and telephone number of the caller. This is necessary in the event that the caller is somehow disconnected. A person who is experiencing a dental emergency should be seen immediately. It is essential to remain calm and reassuring and to give the patient appropriate instructions until he or she arrives at the dental office. If there is any doubt about handling emergency situations, written protocols and rehearsal of emergency procedures are helpful to all dental team members.

LEGAL ISSUES

Taking note of highlights during telephone conversations is courteous and could provide the dentist with legal protection if the information is recorded accurately and concisely in a telephone log. Calls that have clinical significance should be recorded in the patient's chart.

Precautions can be taken to avoid exposure to legal risk by taking the time to improve the existing telephone system and train new staff members in appropriate telephone procedures. Written guidelines delineating responsibilities can also be helpful to ensure that every one is clear about his or her role in telephone communications. Systems should be evaluated regularly to maintain the quality of care and continual improvement.

The dental office administrator should never attempt to diagnose, especially over the telephone. The dentist is the only person who can legally diagnose and treat patients. Improper advice given over the telephone can expose the dentist to unnecessary legal risk.

EQUIPMENT AND TECHNOLOGY

Telecommunications technology is advancing at a rapid pace and creating a faster, more efficient flow of information. The dental office administrator must be familiar with the most current technologies available. Most telecommunications companies are willing to demonstrate their equipment and provide training to staff members. The cost of any new equipment must be justified by improved efficiency and service to patients.

The dental office administrator should learn how to use all of the business equipment to its best advantage. Technology should be used as a tool to increase efficiency, not to slow down productivity. It is

TABLE 9.2 TELEPHONE DECISION GUIDELINES FOR DENTAL DISCOMFORT

QUESTION	NEEDS TO SEE DENTIST IF...	EMERGENCY OR URGENCY
How long have you been experiencing the discomfort?	Rapid onset and acute pain.	Emergency.
	Slow onset, dull pain	Urgency.
Can you describe the discomfort?	Acute pain, localized.	Emergency.
	Dull ache, nonspecific location.	Urgency.
Do you experience sensitivity to hot or cold? If so, which is more severe?	Sensitivity to heat.	Can be an emergency (possible abscess).
	Sensitivity to cold.	Usually an urgency.
Do you have a fever?	Yes.	Emergency. A fever is a normal response to inflammation.
	No.	Urgency.
Is there any swelling?	Yes, with sudden onset.	Emergency.
	No.	Urgency.
Has there been recent trauma, such as a blow to the mouth?	Yes, if so, describe.	Emergency.
	No.	Urgency.
Is there any bleeding? If so, how much?	Yes, extensive.	Emergency.
	Gums bleed when brushing.	Urgency.

important to maintain a positive attitude toward the use of new technologies and to encourage other staff members to do the same. The telephone is one of the most important pieces of equipment in the dental office and it has a profound effect on the success of the practice.

The telephone system will most likely have a minimum of two incoming lines and a private line for outgoing calls. Incoming calls should be answered on the second or third ring. This allows the caller and the receiver of the call time to prepare for the call. Outgoing calls should be made on the private line to keep the incoming lines open as much as possible.

An answering machine or service should be used when the office is closed. It is important to provide 24-hour access to dental care, particularly emergency care. Instructions for after-hours emergency callers should include the name and number of the dentist on call (if available) or directions to proceed to the emergency department of the local hospital. Some dentists prefer to leave their home number for emergency purposes. It is also a courtesy to the caller to state the regular office hours and times for appointments.

Voice Mail

Voice mail provides a convenient method of leaving messages for patients. If the dental office has a voice mail system, it should not be used as a method to screen incoming calls. Callers prefer to speak to responsive human beings and not machines. Some important calls may be missed if the caller is reluctant to use voice mail.

Electronic Mail

Electronic mail (e-mail) is a method of communication that is passed along telephone lines through a modem. The use of e-mail should be limited in a clinical setting as it does not always ensure privacy and, therefore, may intrude on patient confidentiality.

The Hold Button

It will be necessary from time to time to place an incoming caller on hold, possibly to respond to another caller or speak to a dental team member. When it is necessary to place someone on hold, first ask the caller if he or she is able to hold. If it is an emergency, the caller will identify it as such. If it is acceptable to put the caller on hold, remember to get back soon. Thirty seconds on hold can feel much longer to the caller. Ask if the caller would prefer to be called back if it appears that the response will take some time.

An internal communication system may include hands-free paging for communication with the dentist. This feature allows the dentist to communicate important information without interrupting clinical procedures.

TELEPHONE SYSTEM MANAGEMENT

A system of time management will enable the dental office administrator to use the telephone as a valuable business tool. It is helpful if you try to keep incoming lines clear during peak hours, usually between 10:00 a.m. and 2:00 p.m. Patients who wish to make appointments can be instructed to call outside of peak hours to ensure that their calls receive priority treatment.

Personal calls should be avoided if possible. From time to time, a situation may arise that requires a personal call to be taken during business hours. Families of staff members should be encouraged to call during nonpeak hours and to limit personal calls to urgent matters only. Employers do not look favourably on staff members taking too many personal calls.

Outgoing calls for continuing care, collection, appointment confirmation, and treatment follow-up are most successful around the dinner hour. Care should be taken, however, to apologize politely for the interruption. Plan ahead for these outgoing calls and get to the point as quickly as possible after the appropriate greeting and introduction.

Some offices may establish a time for all outgoing administrative calls to be made. Administrative time should never interfere with the productivity of the practice. Therefore, time provided for this purpose should not be when patients are in treatment.

Collection Calls

Calls to collect money can be the most awkward and negative of the outgoing calls you must make, and they should be handled with tact. Collection calls should be made in a private setting, away from other patients who may be listening. The confidentiality of financial information is just as important as that of clinical records. Patients may experience anxiety when reminded of an outstanding account and may have a negative reaction. The dental office administrator must remember not to take this type of reaction personally and should handle the situation with compassion. Uncomfortable situations can be avoided by establishing firm but fair financial policies and educating patients that payment is expected at the time of service.

The dental office administrator should select a day and time when there would be the fewest distractions. A later hour of the day is preferred for collection calls because if they do generate anxiety, it will not affect other patients.

Continuing Care Calls

Repeat business is the backbone of any successful organization. Continuing care calls are the bread and butter of the dental practice. To take advantage of the most favourable time to reach people during the dinner hour, someone would be calling patients between 5:00 and

7:00 p.m. Whoever makes these calls should be very familiar with the appointment scheduling system. It is helpful to have a list of school holidays available as they can be the most productive times in a dental office. It is important to have a positive attitude about ongoing care and to reinforce the idea that regular visits to the dentist can help to avoid costly and uncomfortable treatment.

Follow-Up Calls

Patients who have had extensive dental treatment find it comforting to receive a telephone call from the dental office to see how they are feeling. These calls should be reserved for patients who have had extensive work, such as root canal therapy or major restorative dentistry. Unnecessary calls can alarm patients, making them feel that something went wrong. Letting them know that they are cared for reinforces their loyalty and commitment to the dental office.

Angry Callers

Handling angry callers requires patience and tact. Once again, it is important for the dental office administrator not to take it personally. The most important thing to remember is that patients in this state are usually angry at a situation out of their control. Acknowledging their feelings and allowing them to vent will help them regain control of the situation by recapturing their composure. If at some point there is a positive statement, then it is an appropriate time to cut in. It is absolutely essential that the dental office administrator remains calm and tries to separate the person from the situation. Keep the problem in focus and avoid overly emotional reactions.

The dental office administrator should never raise his or her voice or use profanity. Avoid phrases that will antagonize and provoke anger. It may be necessary to refer the call to the dentist if the situation becomes unmanageable. It is important to follow up with angry callers.

Taking Messages

It is important to take phone messages for others as efficiently as you would like them taken for you. Taking clear messages and delivering them to the appropriate person is a vital aspect of dental office administration. Various forms for taking messages and recording detailed information are available (see Exhibit 9.1).

A simple telephone message slip is shown in Exhibit 9.2.

EXHIBIT 9.1 MESSAGE INFORMATION FORMS

DATE	TIME	CALLER	AREA CODE	TELEPHONE NUMBER	CALL FOR	MESSAGE SLIP NUMBER

HEALTH CARE TELEPHONE MESSAGE LOG FROM: _____ DATE TO: _____ DATE

DATE	TIME	CALLER	AREA CODE	TELEPHONE NUMBER	CALL FOR	MESSAGE SLIP NUMBER
	AM PM					1
	AM PM					2
	AM PM					3
	AM PM					4
	AM PM					
	AM PM					

DATE	TIME	CALLER	AREA CODE	TELEPHONE NUMBER	CALL FOR	MESSAGE SLIP NUMBER

❑ Please Call ❑ Urgent ❑ Professional ❑ Other _____   Patient's Name

❑ Will Call Back ❑ Not Urgent ❑ Rx Renewal _____   **1243**

Complaint or Message

Diagnosis

Treatment Recommended

Presently taking medication? ❑ Yes ❑ No

Allergies?

MESSAGE TAKEN BY	CALL - BACK TIMES AVAIL	ALTERNATE PHONE NUMBER	HANDLED BY	DATE	TIME
					AM PM
	AM PM					17
	AM PM					18
	AM PM					19
	AM PM					20
	AM PM					21
	AM PM					22
	AM PM					23
	AM PM					24
	AM PM					25

NOTE LINE #	ADDITIONAL COMMENTS

Used with permission by Safeguard Business Systems, Inc., Fort Washington, PA 19034

EXHIBIT 9.2 **TELEPHONE MESSAGE SLIP**

TELEPHONE MESSAGE

To:_____

Date: _____

WHILE YOU WERE OUT

From: _____

Of: _____

Phone: _____

Message:_____

_____

_____

_____

Signed: _____

The person receiving the message must be able to read and interpret it at a glance. Messages should contain the following essential facts:

- name and telephone number of the caller
- date and time of the call
- message including what action needs to be taken
- name of the person who took the message

A message is of no value if it is incomplete or illegible. The proper recording of telephone messages can provide the dental office with legal protection also. Therefore, care must be taken to print clearly to ensure that the message will not be subject to misinterpretation.

Screening Calls

It is important not to interrupt the dentist or any of the clinical staff during clinical procedures except for an absolute emergency. Screening calls is a time saver and support service for the dentist. The dental office administrator should be courteous and collect all necessary information, while reassuring the caller that the message will be treated as a priority and will reach the dentist immediately. Dental salespeople are well trained to get through the protective screening process. Be firm but courteous when dealing with them.

ASSIGNMENT

1. Briefly describe how you would handle the following incoming telephone calls:
   a. Mrs. Smith has broken a tooth and needs to see the dentist right away. She is experiencing a great deal of discomfort and the schedule is completely filled.
   b. Mr. Jones calls saying his son has just been hit in the mouth with a hockey puck and is bleeding profusely. He cannot tell if any teeth are broken.
   c. Mr. Green has had a dull, nagging toothache for about a week and would like it to be fixed today because he is going away for the weekend.

2. Replace the following statements with more positive ones:
   "The dentist is running late ... "
   "The dentist is tied up with a patient ... "
   "The treatment is not painful ... "
   "The dentist may have to pull the tooth out ..."
   "We have had a cancellation today ... "

3. Create a script for a fictitious dental office and tape record how you would answer an incoming call and/or leave a message on an answering machine. Ask a class member to honestly evaluate your voice quality using the following questions:
   a. Did you answer promptly and greet the caller pleasantly?
   b. Did you identify the office and yourself properly and show that you will take responsibility for the call?
   c. Did you give the regular office hours?
   d. Did you provide clear instructions if it was an emergency call?
   e. Did you speak clearly?

CHAPTER TEN

RECALL SYSTEMS

OBJECTIVE

At the end of this chapter, the student will be able to identify and describe the following: The importance of continuing care appointments and follow-up, various types of recall systems, and how to establish an effective recall system.

TOPICS

- the purpose of the recall appointment
- what works and what does not
- types of recall systems
- understanding the patient's attitudes toward health care
- educating patients on the importance of preventive care
- value of follow-up

CONTINUING CARE

One of the most crucial elements for practice growth and stability is an effective recall or continuous care system. Repeat business is the vital link between success and failure. The patients in a dental office are the clients or "customers," and it is important to keep the customer coming back. It is the job of the dental team to encourage patients to return to the practice for continuous treatment.

Dentists often prefer to use the term "continuing care appointment" or "recare appointment" rather than "recall." It is important to realize that this is the lifeline of a dental practice. The key to a successful health care program is prevention of illness or disease. Dental disease is easily prevented and a preventive care program will ultimately save patients time, money, and discomfort. Making patients aware that the recall system is a plan for ongoing preventive dental care and maintenance enhances their understanding and encourages cooperation in this collaborative effort.

A recall system has to be continually maintained. Otherwise, the financial productivity of the practice will begin to suffer and growth will not occur.

PATIENT ATTITUDES TOWARD HEALTH CARE

The success of any recall system depends on how the patient feels about returning to the practice. Motivating a patient to return can be challenging. Each person is an individual with a complex structure of needs.

Many successful dental office administrators have found that their success is at least partly due to the continuous positive reinforcement about health care that is reflected throughout the office by every staff member. Patients need to be reassured that they have made a good decision and have invested their health care dollars wisely. Dental care is an investment in one's own health. Patients must be willing to invest their time and money to achieve optimum dental health. Not all patients are fortunate enough to be covered by dental insurance. Those who aren't need to feel that their investment is worthwhile. Generally speaking, most people are willing to invest in their health care if they truly understand the value of the service.

People generally would like to live longer, feel better, and look great. A beautiful, healthy smile is aesthetically pleasing and reflects this philosophy. The smile is one of the most powerful methods of human communication, as it crosses all barriers of language or culture. It indicates acceptance and trust to the receiver. As an added benefit, a smile makes the person smiling feel good also.

Positive motivation, courtesy, and respect will encourage patients to return to the practice and also to refer their friends and relatives. Patients need to be motivated to accept responsibility for their own dental health and then to receive positive reinforcement that this is a wise decision.

WHY IS A RECALL SYSTEM IMPORTANT TO THE PATIENT?

Patients need to know that the dentist and the dental team care about their dental health. Patients who have no further contact with the office after the first visit will feel that the dental staff really do not care about their dental health and will be less likely to return.

It is important to recognize and acknowledge patients as individuals and make them feel that they are important. Their repeat business and continued loyalty will not be gained until they feel valued as patients and human beings.

One method of acknowledging a patient's uniqueness is to use his or her name. It is appropriate to use a patient's last name and title, such as Mr. Jones, Mrs. Smith, etc. If the patient prefers that the dental team use his or her first name, then it is acceptable to do so. This simple act allows the patient to feel acknowledged as a person and not a number. Many health care providers are recognizing the importance of treating the whole patient and not just an illness.

TYPES OF RECALL SYSTEMS

There are a variety of systems available to the dental office administrator. The methods presented represent guidelines only, as none of the methods is perfect. The dental office administrator should decide which method, or combination of methods, is best suited for the practice, accurately representing its image and philosophy.

Telephone System

The telephone system is one of the most effective recall systems, although it can be time-consuming. Many large dental practices will hire someone who has the primary responsibility of recalling patients. The administrators of such practices recognize the importance of an effective system and are willing to invest in training employees to become recall specialists. The telephone calling system is an effective practice builder, providing the patient with human contact. Many patients appreciate the telephone call to remind them that they are due for their appointment and depend on that reminder.

One of the main disadvantages of this system is that patients may not be at home or may not wish to be disturbed, particularly at their workplace. One of the best times to call patients is during the dinner hours (between 5:00 and 7:00 p.m.). Many people are home at that time, but they may not appreciate being disturbed, so tact and good manners should be exercised.

Another disadvantage of the telephone calling system is the time it takes. The office administrator may find it difficult to find the time to call patients and schedule their appointments, along with the various other duties that he or she is responsible for. Ideally, this task can be delegated to someone whose primary responsibility is to recall patients on a regular basis.

The latter is recommended, as the recall procedure is so vital to the success of the dental practice. In addition to having responsibility for recall appointments, this person could also call patients to confirm appointments, receive incoming calls, and so on.

A telephone recall system will involve the following functions:

1. The office administrator pulls all of the charts for patients who are due for recall appointments. The Mardan charting system provides an effective system of identification using colour coded tabs inserted in the month that the appointment is due.

2. When the call is made to the patient, it is recorded on the front of the chart cover. If the patient is not available, the chart will be held out until contact can be made. After three or four attempts at calling, a card should be sent to the patient, the colour of the tab changed and moved to the next month. Attempts to contact the patient will then be deferred until the following month.

3. When the appointment has been set, the date is recorded on the front of the chart cover and the chart refiled.

4. When the current month's calls have been completed, the administration will pull the charts for the next month.

It is extremely important that the dental office administrator check the date of the last recall appointment. As most dental insurance policies limit the frequency of preventive recall appointments, the patient may not be covered by dental insurance if the next appointment date is prior to the limitation requirement, even by one day. In addition, it is illegal to change the date on a claim form; the date of the treatment must match the date on the chart. It is helpful if recall appointment entries are made in different colours within the chart.

Not all insurance companies provide coverage for six-month recalls. Many carriers have reduced the frequency to nine months. Check coverage limitations with the patient and take the extra time to check the date of the last recall on the chart.

Mail System

The mail system consists of mailing patients a recall card or letter. The card will remind the patient that an appointment is due and request that he or she call the office. The responsibility for making the appointment is placed on the patient. The advantage of this system is that it is less time-consuming initially than the telephone system. Cards can be selected that have catchy phrases and pictures, or they may contain the logo of the dental office.

One of the disadvantages of the mail system is that it is expensive because of increasing postage costs as well as the cost of printing the cards. It is also very easy to ignore a card or letter compared to a personal telephone call. A patient may procrastinate about scheduling the appointment; thus, the dental office will not receive an immediate response.

The mail system requires more follow-up on the part of the office administrator and control of the recall appointments is left up to the patients. There is a risk that patients will become lost in the system.

The mechanics of the mail system are similar to the telephone system and are as follows:

1. The office administrator will pull all of the charts for patients who are due for recall appointments.
2. A recall card should be completed for each and the date sent recorded on the front of the chart cover. Sometimes the card may have a carbon copy attached, which can be placed in the file and removed after the patient has made the appointment.
3. When the appointment has been scheduled, the date is recorded on the front of the chart cover and the chart refiled.
4. When the current month has been completed, charts are pulled for the next month.

Continuous Appointment System

The continuous appointment system is sometimes referred to as the advanced appointment system. When the patient completes an appointment, an advance appointment for six or nine months in the future is scheduled at that time. This system saves the administrator a great deal of time as there is no further direct contact with the patient until the next appointment. When appointments are scheduled six months in advance, the dental office can make an accurate prediction of financial activity over the coming months.

Although this system appears to be ideal, it is vulnerable to many variables, such as the dentist or hygienist becoming ill or leaving the practice. It also limits the number of openings available in the hygiene schedule for new patients. Patients may be reluctant to schedule six months in advance because they often do not know what they will be doing that far ahead. Patients should be encouraged to make appointments knowing that they can be changed if necessary, but reminded of office policy requiring advance notice of changes.

The mechanics of the continuous appointment system are as follows:

1. When the current course of treatment is completed, the patient is told that the dentist has requested to see him or her again and asked to schedule the next appointment.
2. Once a convenient appointment is made, the date and time is repeated to the patient.
3. As the appointment is made, an appointment card is completed and handed to the patient. This provides the patient with a tangible reminder to return to the practice.
4. The patient should be asked if he or she prefers a telephone call to confirm the appointment in advance. Some patients pride themselves on having an excellent memory and do not appreciate a reminder call. If the patient does not wish to be called, note that on the schedule. The office administrator will save time if some calls are not needed.
5. If the patient requires a confirmation call, file a reminder two days in advance of the appointment and call to confirm it.

Combination Recall System

A recall system that has proven to be effective is one that incorporates all three systems. The combination system reduces the number of "no shows" or patients forgetting about their appointments.

The combination system is based primarily on the advanced booking system, in that patients are encouraged to schedule future appointments, usually six months in advance. Once again, the patient is reassured that he or she will be called in advance as a reminder and will have an opportunity to reschedule if necessary.

When the appointment is made, the patient is asked to complete a postcard with his or her name and address. The date and time of the appointment will be filled in on the postcard, much like an appointment card. The post card will then be filed in the month previous to the appointment (e.g., if the appointment is scheduled for May, the card will be filed under April). At the beginning of each month, all of the filed cards are mailed out. This method is extremely effective because people do not usually receive mail addressed to themselves in their own handwriting. It will attract attention and remind patients of the commitment they made to return for the recall appointment, while once again reinforcing the dental office's cancellation policy.

Patients who still wish to be reminded should be called two days in advance. Indicate on the schedule appointments made six months earlier that require confirmation.

The mechanics of the combination recall system are as follows:

1. When the patient has completed a course of treatment, you will tell him or her that the doctor has asked for a future appointment.
2. As the appointment is being made, have the patient personally address a postcard. Write the date and time of the appointment on the postcard.
3. Always repeat the date and time to the patient.
4. Ask if the patient prefers to be called to confirm the appointment.
5. If the patient requires a confirmation call, file a reminder two days in advance of the appointment and call to confirm it.
6. File the postcard in the month previous to the appointment. This allows the patient an entire month to reschedule if necessary.

The combination recall system can save the dental office administrator an enormous amount of time and ensure that the patient is effectively recalled. A well-organized and dedicated administrator will find this system to be easy to use as it shares the responsibility between the patient and the dental office.

Computerized Recall Systems

A computer is extremely valuable to a recall system. Although dental software packages differ somewhat in design, most will include a recall reminder or "tickler" system. Once recall due dates are entered into patient records, a report can be generated each day with a list of patients who are due for their appointments. The list can be used as a reminder to you to follow up with these patients.

With a computerized list, the dental office administrator can organize every day to include recall and confirmation calls. Although some days will be busier than others, they will be more manageable when the workload is distributed throughout the year.

Each of the recall systems has clear advantages and disadvantages. A combination of systems might be appropriate for the needs of your office. The objective of each system is to encourage repeat business and preventive health care. Regardless of which recall system is chosen, once it is established, regular follow-up and maintenance is crucial for the ongoing success of the practice.

ASSIGNMENT

1. When should the patient be recalled to the practice?
2. Based on the information that you studied in this chapter, which recall system or combination system would you recommend and why?
3. Why are recalls crucial to the success of a dental practice?
4. When do you feel is the best time to call patients when using the telephone recall system? Why?
5. When do you think that you should not call patients? Why?
6. Design a recall card or letter that will encourage patients to schedule their appointments.

CHAPTER ELEVEN

ACCOUNTS RECEIVABLE

OBJECTIVE

At the end of this chapter, the student will be able to identify and describe the following: How to record daily financial transactions, balance the daysheet, establish and maintain a petty cash system, handle postdated cheques, cash, and credit card payments, collect payment at the time of service, make financial arrangements that are in keeping with office policy, and keep accounts receivable low while increasing productivity.

TOPICS

- bookkeeping systems
- the One Write accounting system
- debits, credits, and running balances
- ledger cards
- payments (credit cards, postdated cheques, cash)
- petty cash
- collections
- financial arrangements
- monthly statements
- reversals, adjustments, and write-offs
- error detection, helpful hints

IMPORTANCE OF FINANCIAL CONTROL

Dentistry is a business. All successful businesses require strong management and control of financial records. A well-organized dental office administrator can help to reduce fees paid to accounting services by maintaining accurate, complete, and up-to-date records.

Dentists generally use accounting services to prepare their financial statements and summarize the financial records for tax purposes. The accountant works hand in hand with the dental office administrator to provide financial and legal protection for the dentist. The accountant, however, should not be required to take care of basic bookkeeping that can be done at the dental office. It is not cost effective to have the accounting office do bookkeeping. This is the responsibility of the administrator.

Financial records should be maintained separately from clinical records. Proper care and maintenance of the financial records can save time, reduce the chances of revenue being lost, and protect the dental office against unnecessary legal problems. Financial information is **highly confidential**, whether it is the patient's information or the dentist's. Every effort should be made to protect the confidentiality of these records. The dental office administrator is responsible for the appropriate handling of all money received in the practice and the accurate recording of all transactions.

Accounting is the classifying, recording, and summarizing of all financial transactions. Bookkeeping is the recording part of this process. There are two types of bookkeeping systems used in a dental office:

1. Accounts Receivable (A/R)
2. Accounts Payable (A/P)

The accounts receivable represent all charges, payments, and outstanding balances **owed to** the practice. Accounts payable represent all money **owed by** the practice. This chapter deals with the accounts receivable bookkeeping system only.

Many dental offices have computer systems that record and calculate the accounts receivable transactions. Computerized tracking of accounts receivable allows the dentist, the administrator, and the accounting service instant access to important financial information, such as the aged accounts receivable list.

It is important to understand bookkeeping entries on a manual system in order to know how to make account adjustments electronically. A solid understanding of the basic principles of bookkeeping, along with good mathematical skills, forms the foundation of accurate record keeping.

EXHIBIT 11.1 AGED RECEIVABLES—PATIENTS

For:03/MAR/95
03:16p

Family Dental Centre
For Practice: ?

P/D Range: 00001 – 00500   Days Owing: 0   Balances Over 0.00   Last Statement more than 0 days ago

PID	Name	0–29	30–59	60–89	90–119	120+	Last Pmt	Curr Bal.	Ins Plan	Asngd?	Phone	Pat Dnt
	Balances Owing:											
00150	ALLISON, Mrs. Mildred	227.63					29/JAN/95	227.63	ABEL	Y	(905)433–5400	H
00115	ASHBERRY, Mrs. Edna	205.20					PD 51.00	205.20	ABEL	Y	(905)354–5444	L
00116	ASHBERRY, Mr. Kal W.	80.00					PD 80.00	80.00	GREAT	N	(905)443–6509	H
00190	BALL, Mr. Derrick A.	89.00					PD 89.00	89.00	MUTUA	N	(905)343–6550	H
00227	BERRY, Mrs. Ellen		702.13				07/NOV/94	702.13	ODA	Y	(905)537–3344	C
00318	BLAKE, Mr. Dave D. Sr.	75.00					PD 75.00	75.00	GREAT	N	(416)343-5634	L
00290	BOLTON, Mrs. Kathleen	310.00					PD 10.00	310.00			(905)342–6151	H
00346	BRAZIER, Mrs. Wendy					646.95	01/SEP/94	646.95			(905)663–1047	H
	see Lloyd or Pat re: pmt											
00382	BROOKS, Mrs. Sally	140.00					28/NOV/94	140.00	BLUE +	N	(905)389–4011	H
	will have Veronica send pmt											
00417	BROWN, Mrs. Brenda	493.00					PD 38.00	493.00	ABEL	Y	(905)389–6333	H
00461	BUCKLEY, Mr. Bill	253.14	72.12				30/NOV/94	325.26			(905)333–2176	H
00296	DOVEY, Mrs. Debra	135.00					01/JUN/94	135.00	SUNLIF	N	(905)423–1055	H
00271	FAWCETT, Mrs. Lori	634.00					28/NOV/94	634.00	EMPIRE	N	(416)664--4438	L
	will drop pmt off PJ											
00449	GUTHRIE, Mr. Arlo A.	54.20	11.67			13.55	21/SEP/94	79.42	ABEL	Y	(416)359–2084	L
	(BUD)											
00220	HALSTEAD, Mr. Larry	176.00					PD 161.00	176.00	BLUE +	N	(905)484–5587	L
00373	PRINDLE, Mr. Rob R.	347.00				450.00	29/NOV/94	797.00	ABEL	Y	(905)533–6247	H
	see notesheet re: visa pmts											
00490	TOFFOLO, Mr. Mark W.	80.39					18/OCT/94	80.39	ODA	Y	(905)534–6716	L
	Totals for Balances Owing:	3299.56	785.92	0.00	0.00	1110.50	1104.00	5195.98				
		63.5%	15.1%	0.0%	0.0%	21.4%	21.2%	100.0%				
	Collection Balances:											
00177	AMBROSE, Mr. David					20.00		20.00			(416)376–3344	H
	N.S.F. SERVICE CHARGE OUTSTANDING											
00264	BAKER, Mrs. Pamela					75.00	27/JUL/94	75.00	ODA	Y	(416)842-3457	
	OUTSTANDING NO SHOW FEES EIGHT APPOINTMENTS											
00082	FARRONE, Miss Joan					25.00		25.00			(905)389–1354	C
	OUTSTANDING NO SHOW CHARGE											
00479	WYNETTE, Ms. Tammy					30.00	31/DEC/93	30.00	ODA	Y	(416)534–7687	H
	OUTSTANDING NO SHOW CHARGE											
	Totals for Collection Accts:	0.00	0.00	0.00	0.00	150.00		150.00				
		0.0%	0.0%	0.0%	0.0%	100.0%		100.0%				
	Totals for All Balances:	3299.56	785.92	0.00	0.00	1260.50	1104.00	5345.98				
		61.7%	14.7%	0.0%	0.0%	23.6%	20.7%	100.0%				

Sample provided by ABEL Computers Ltd., Burlington, Ontario.

THE ONE WRITE BOOKKEEPING SYSTEM

One very effective and widely used manual bookkeeping system is the One Write pegboard system, which is designed and distributed by Safeguard Business Systems. The principle of the One Write system is to record the financial transaction on three forms simultaneously. Through the interleaving of the daily journal page, the patient ledger card, and a receipt, all the necessary financial records for each patient visit are completed by writing the information just once.

The following information is recorded on all three records:

- name of patient
- code for treatment provided
- charges made to the account
- payments received
- outstanding balance
- account adjustments

Writing the financial transaction only once helps to ensure the accuracy of the entry on all records.

LEAFLET RECEIPTS

The receipts that are given to patients have multiple functions. They act as charge slips to record the fee charged and payment made. They can be used as "walk-out" statements for patients who wish to mail payments in at a later time. The receipts can be used to transmit fee information from the treatment area to the business office, thus acting as communication slips. They are also an important part of the audit trail to verify that the transactions are recorded for every patient seen during the day.

The receipt pages are arranged as leaflets, numbered sequentially. The administrator will write the name of each patient on a separate leaflet at the beginning of the day. If a slip is left unaccounted for at the end of the day, this usually indicates that charges were not posted for that patient. An incomplete slip will alert the dental office administrator to verify whether the patient was seen in the office that day. The receipt numbers are also recorded on the daily journal page. All numbers must be accounted for.

EXHIBIT 11.2 ONE WRITE BOOKKEEPING SYSTEM

RECORD OF CHARGES AND RECEIPTS

RECEIPT NUMBER	DATE	DESCRIPTION - CODE	CHARGE	PAYMENT	BALANCE	✓	PREVIOUS BALANCE	NAME		1	2
									1		
									2		
									3		
									4		
									5		
									6		
									7		
									8		
									9		
									10		

RECEIPT NUMBER	DATE	DESCRIPTION - CODE	CHARGE	PAYMENT	CURRENT BALANCE	PREVIOUS BALANCE	NAME

YOU PAID THIS AMOUNT ↗

DR. LORNE NEWTON
Dental Surgeon
TOWNLEY DENTAL OFFICE
7380 McCOWAN RD., UNIT 1 MARKHAM, ONT. L3S 3H8
TELEPHONE: 479-7443

Please present this slip to admitting office before leaving.

SERVICES RENDERED   **FEE**

A1 – One Surface Silver Restoration
A2 – Two Surface Silver Restoration
A3 – Three Surface Silver Restoration
AN – Analgesia
BR – Bridge
CF – Composite Resin Filling (White)

C – Crown
CX – Complicated Extraction
DM – Diagnostic Models
DR – Denture Repair or Reline
ET – Emergency Treatment
EX – Examination and Diagnosis
EXT – Extraction
FD – Full Denture

FL – Fluoride Treatment
FMS – Full Mouth X-Ray Survey
L – Lab. Charge
MA – Missed Appointment
OC – Bite Correction
OHI – Oral Hygiene Instruction
OR – Orthodontic Treatment
P – Pin Reinforcement
P & C – Post & Core

PD – Partial Denture
PU – Pulpotomy
PRO – Prophylaxis
PT – Gum Disease Tx
PX – Panoramic X-Ray
RCT – Root Canal Therapy
ROA – Received on Account
RX – Recall Examination
S – Scaling
SM – Space Maintainer
TF – Treatment Filling
X – X-Rays

RECEIVED PAYMENT ....

TOTAL $

NEXT APPOINTMENT .... AT ....
Date   Time

1447	PLEASE RETAIN: This is the only completely itemized statement you will receive. The amount shown in the payment column may be for income tax purposes.	1447	NEXT APPOINTMENT
1448	PLEASE RETAIN: This is the only completely itemized statement you will receive. The amount shown in the payment column may be for income tax purposes.	1448	NEXT APPOINTMENT
1449	PLEASE RETAIN: This is the only completely itemized statement you will receive. The amount shown in the payment column may be for income tax purposes.	1449	NEXT APPOINTMENT
1450	PLEASE RETAIN: This is the only completely itemized statement you will receive. The amount shown in the payment column may be for income tax purposes.	1450	NEXT APPOINTMENT

(rows 11–30)

COLUMN A	COLUMN B	COLUMN C	COLUMN D	TOTALS

▲ ALL RECEIPTS MUST BE IN NUMERICAL ORDER

PROOF OF POSTING	ACCOUNTS RECEIVABLE CONTROL	OPENING CASH ON HAND	DAILY CASH SUMMARY	
COLUMN D TOTAL: _____	A/R BAL. FWD.: _____	AT BEGINNING OF DAY $ _____		CASH PAID OUT $ _____
"+" COLUMN A TOTAL: _____	"+" COLUMN A: _____	CASH REC'D DURING DAY $ _____		BANK DEPOSITS $ _____
SUB TOTAL: _____	SUB TOTAL: _____	TOTAL $ _____		CLOSING CASH ON HAND $ _____
"–" COLUMN B TOTAL: _____	"–" COLUMN B: _____	CASH LONG $ _____		TOTAL $ _____
"=" COLUMN C TOTAL: _____	PRESENT A/R BAL.: _____	TOTAL $ _____		CASH SHORT $ _____
				TOTAL $ _____

DATE
PAGE NO.

Used with permission by Safeguard Business Systems, Inc., Fort Washington, PA 19034

EXHIBIT 11.3 **PATIENT RECEIPT FORM**

RECEIPT NUMBER	DATE	DESCRIPTION · CODE	CHARGE	PAYMENT	CURRENT BALANCE

YOU PAID THIS AMOUNT⎯⎯⎯⎯⎯⎯⎯⎯↑

AM — 1,2,3, etc. Surfaces Amalgam Restoration	D — Dentures	G — Gold Inlay	PRO — Prophylaxis
BR — Bridge	DR — Denture Reline	NC — No Charge	PT — Periodontal Treatment
CN — Crown	ET — Endodontic Therapy	O — Orthodontic Treatment	ROA — Received on Account
CR — Composite Restoration	EX — Examination	OHI — Oral Hygiene Instruction	SM — Space Maintainer
CX — Complete Series X-Rays	EXT — Extraction	PD — Partial Denture	TF — Temporary Filling
	FA — Failed Appointment		X — X-Ray
	FT — Fluoride Treatment		

RECEIVED PAYMENT ....

NEXT APPOINTMENT .... AT ....
                                                Date   Time

Used with permission by Safeguard Business Systems, Inc., Fort Washington, PA 19034

The leaflet receipts also provide a legend of codes for a variety of dental services. Using the codes will help to record accurately the types of services provided in a very limited space, usually one line. For example,

AM—indicates an amalgam filling

EX—indicates an examination

X—indicates that an x-ray was taken

THE LEDGER CARD

The ledger card is a record that shows charges, payments, and balances owed for each patient or family. It may also include coded and itemized information concerning services rendered. It is essential to press firmly when recording transactions on the ledger card so that the information is easy to read and understand. All fees and payments for professional treatment are posted daily to the ledger card.

EXHIBIT 11.4 **LEDGER CARD**

Mrs. Jane
John Jr.
123 Main St.   H: 5551212
City, Province   W: 5552233 (Mr.)
Postal Code

NUMBER	DATE	DESCRIPTION	CHARGE		PAYMENT		CURRENT BALANCE	
0001	07/07	Ama, 1,6, MOD (Mr)	87	50	87	50	0	

SAFEGUARD BUSINESS SYSTEMS Form No. ARL-M5-4-BF
THO USA

PLEASE PAY LAST AMOUNT IN BALANCE COLUMN ➜

Used with permission by Safeguard Business Systems, Inc., Fort Washington, PA 19034

The ledger card should include as much information as possible on each family. Family accounts are addressed to the person responsible for the account. Therefore, all ledger cards have the name and complete address, including postal code, neatly recorded in the appropriate space.

Notes to indicate whether the family has dental insurance and a summary of the plan coverage can be included on the ledger card. Care should be taken to code this information clearly and concisely to avoid making the card appear cluttered.

For example, GWL R-100, M-50, O-50 indicates that the patient has insurance coverage under Great West Life. The program design is 100 percent for routine care, 50 percent coverage for major restorative treatment (such as crowns, bridges, and dentures), and 50 percent for orthodontics. Never write derogatory remarks about a patient on the ledger card, such as "bad account" or "always late."

Charges to patients' accounts are called debits, and payments made are credits. If there is a balance owing on a patient's account, the account has a debit balance.

Ledger cards should be stored in a ledger card tray. This is often referred to as a vertical file. The ledger card tray is metal and allows easy expansion when in use. At night the tray should be tightened to keep the ledger cards tightly packed. This will provide a small degree of protection in the event of a fire, as tightly packed paper does not burn as quickly. The best protection against fire, however, is storage in a fireproof cabinet or safe.

The front of the ledger tray will contain the accounts receivable, in other words, the cards for all the patients who owe money to the practice. When an account is paid in full, the ledger card can then be filed alphabetically at the back of the ledger tray.

A common error that is easily made with ledger cards is to file them with patient charts. **Remember to keep financial and clinical information separate.** It is very easy to stand a ledger card upright in the chart cover while speaking with a patient concerning his or her account. If that card accidentally gets filed with the chart, the accounts receivable will not balance at the end of the month. It will cost the dental practice time and money to recover the misplaced ledger card.

Posting Daily Entries

1. Pull out the ledger cards for each patient the day ahead, after the appointment has been confirmed.

2. As each patient enters the office, complete the stub portion of the service receipt with the name of the person responsible for the account, as well as the previous balance.

3. Detach the stub and attach it to the patient's chart. This is the communication slip.

4. In the operatory, the dentist will indicate the services rendered, fees (if applicable), and the time for the next appointment.

5. Place the ledger card under the remaining portion of the receipt until it is resting against the pegs and align it so that the carbon strip is directly over the first open line and all forms are lined up vertically.

7. Complete the service receipt: receipt number, date, description (from codes given), patient name, total payment received, and balance owing.

8. Detach the receipt from the pegboard.

9. If payment was received, sign or initial the receipt in the place provided.

10. Staple the stub and receipt together and give them to the patient. If there is an outstanding balance, circle it in red and give the receipt to the patient in a self-addressed payment envelope.

11. Place the ledger card back into the appropriate section of the ledger tray.

THE DAYSHEET

On the daily journal page (or daysheet), the office administrator records entries that identify the financial activity and treatment performed on each patient (see Exhibit 11.2). This is the detailed record of every financial transaction that occurred as a result of professional treatment. Each entry includes

1. patient's name
2. treatment provided
3. charges made
4. payments received
5. balance due
6. adjustments made

The daysheet also provides a system for recording and monitoring the daily clinical productivity and breaking it down according to the service provider. The right side of the daysheet contains columns that are used for production breakdown, information that is important for practice analysis. For example, this information may help to determine whether there is a need to hire another full-time or part-time hygienist. These columns also help to record the fees of associate dentists. The accounting service will obtain information about the dentist's income from the daysheet for tax purposes.

In summary, the daysheet is a record of the daily activity in the dental office. The daysheet is set up in columns, which line up exactly with the leaflet receipts and the ledger cards. The columns are as follows:

Column A—Charges All fees charged for professional treatment will be recorded in this column. Account adjustments, write-offs, and courtesy discounts will also be recorded here. The amount of an adjustment or write-off should be surrounded by brackets. The brackets indicate a reversal. The amount in brackets is then subtracted instead of added when totalling the columns.

Column B—Payments All payments received are recorded in this column. The total must match the amount of the bank deposit exactly.

Column C—Current balance The amount that the patient currently owes is recorded here.

Column D—Previous balance This column should be completed first, at the beginning of the day when all of the ledger cards are pulled and the communications slips (or receipt stubs) are prepared. If there is an outstanding balance owing, the amount appears on the communication slip that goes to the treatment room.

At the end of the day all columns should be added up and the totals written at the end of each.

Daily Balancing Procedure

"Proof of posting" is done at the end of the day. The listings on the daily journal page are compared with the appointment book to verify that all patient visits have been entered. These totals represent all of the charges (production), receipts for that day, and the new account balances. The proof of posting section on the daysheet provides a formula to verify the accuracy of all transactions. The formula is as follows:

Previous balance +	Current charges −	Payments received =	Current balance

Using the column totals in this formula will produce the daily balance owing to the practice.

Column D (previous balance)

+ Column A (today's charges—debits)

- Column B (payments received—credits)

= Column C (current balance)

The total of the cash receipts (including cheques and credit card payments) *must* match the amount that is in the cash drawer, which will subsequently be deposited to the bank. The proof of posting section should be completed every day, and any errors must be corrected immediately.

Steps to Balancing

If the daysheet does not balance, try the following:
1. Determine the amount of the difference.
2. Scan the daysheet looking for the amount of the difference.
3. Check all of the adjustments made.
4. Check all amounts recorded in the previous balance column (Column D) with the ledger cards. This column is where many errors occur.
5. Check to see if the amount of the difference is divisible by nine; if so, there could be a transposition of figures. For example, the number 86 could have been recorded instead of 68, or 74 instead of 47, etc.
6. Check each individual posted entry with each ledger card.

Once the daysheet is balanced, the accounts receivable control section can be completed.
1. Bring forward the accounts receivable total from the previous day.
2. Add the charges from the day and subtotal.
3. Subtract the day's payments.
4. Calculate the new accounts receivable control balance.

Total charges and payments are then entered on the monthly summary sheet.

ADVANCE PAYMENTS

Occasionally a patient may wish to make a deposit against future charges, creating a credit balance. This may be done, for example, for crown and bridge or root canal therapy. The payment is noted as follows:

1. Enter the amount paid as a payment on the patient's card and the daysheet.
2. Deduct the payment from the previous balance.
3. If the new balance is a negative figure, show it as a bracketed amount.
4. When subsequent services are performed, reduce the credit balance by the amount of the charge. Enter the charge in the same manner as other charges.

REFUNDS OF CREDIT BALANCES

If a patient has overpaid and a refund is due, enter the amount of the refund as a charge. This amount added to the previous credit balance will bring the patient's balance to nil. Make a notation in the production breakdown column.

BAD DEBTS

When an account balance has to be written off (i.e., sent to a credit bureau or collection service), this amount is deducted from the charges for the day when totalling the daysheet. In the production columns on the daysheet, write an explanation for the bad debt write-off. The accountant will ask about all amounts that are adjusted or written off in the charges column.

On a separate bad debt memo enter the date, name, and amount written off. If money is eventually collected on an account that has been written off, enter the name and the amount as both a charge and a payment, leaving a nil balance.

NSF CHEQUES

NSF means not sufficient funds. On the patient's ledger card and on the daysheet, enter the amount of the returned cheque as a charge again to bring the account back to the balance before the cheque was deducted. Add to the amount the applicable bank charges. Call the patient immediately. When a new cheque is received, enter it in the same manner as other payments. The amount of the new cheque should include the bank charges.

BALANCING THE ACCOUNTS RECEIVABLE

When the daysheet has been balanced and the accounts receivable control completed, the dental office administrator should add up the totals on all of the ledger cards from the front of the ledger tray. The total of the amounts owing on the ledger cards should match the accounts receivable total at that time. It is helpful to use an adding machine that will produce a paper tape. If the accounts receivable balance does not match the total of the ledger cards, follow the steps to balancing listed previously.

Many dental office administrators will incorporate this procedure into the month-end procedures. When it is done more frequently, there is a greater opportunity for controlling and maintaining accurate records. Balancing the accounts receivable at least twice per month is recommended. If errors do occur, it is much easier to go back through the entries made in the past one or two weeks than through an entire month.

FINANCIAL ARRANGEMENTS

Financial arrangements must be made with each patient for whom professional services are performed. Patients should be told of the financial policy of the office and their agreement to the terms secured. All financial arrangements should be made *prior* to treatment except in the case of emergency procedures. Discussion of financial arrangements should be incorporated into each prepared clinical case presentation.

Financial arrangements should be made in privacy and in an unhurried atmosphere with the person who is responsible for the account. These arrangements should be realistic to ensure that the dentist receives appropriate compensation for professional services and that the patient has access to quality health care. A patient's financial status is a very personal and sensitive issue, which should be approached in a caring and professional manner. Try to avoid embarrassing the patient.

Realistic arrangements will take into consideration the payment options available, the patient's ability to pay, and payment preference. The dentist's stated financial policy and sound business management principles must also be considered and applied. The financial arrangements must be equitable to both parties. The dental office administrator should **never prejudge the patient's ability to pay.**

The patient must accept responsibility for his or her own account. All financial agreements should be recorded on the account ledger card or on a written policy agreement. If a contract is signed, the copy is given to the patient and the original is retained with the office records. A written confirmation of the financial discussion helps the administrator recall specific details and protects the practice legally against default on payment.

Methods of Payment

There are many ways in which payment can be made to the dental office. The patient should always be encouraged to pay for the service at the time it is rendered. Some payment options include cheques, postdated cheques, credit cards, or cash. The patient may choose one of these options or may wish to make small regular payments. The dental office administrator should assume that the patient intends to pay for the service performed. Do not ask a patient a question such as, "Would you like to pay for this today?" The reply may be "No." A more appropriate phrasing would be, "How do you intend to take care of your account today? Will that be cash, cheque, postdated cheque, VISA, or Mastercard?"

Be helpful to the patient and offer to make financial arrangements that will be comfortable to both parties. This approach usually results in a more cooperative effort to pay the account.

The fees charged represent a fair return to the dentist for the professional services performed. Many dental office administrators find requesting payment one of their most difficult duties. Practising does help, although it may feel awkward at first. Remember to use eye contact and maintain a pleasant facial expression.

COLLECTION PROCEDURES

Statements

Monthly statements must be professional in appearance and should create a positive impression. They should always be neat and legible and should reflect the professional image of the dental office. Itemized statements help to eliminate misunderstandings about fees.

Statements must be **routinely mailed at the same time each month**. In most offices, it is preferred to have the statements mailed so that patients receive them on or before the first of the month. Some offices prefer to send the statements during the middle of the month so that the dental office statement will not be received at the same time as other monthly statements.

The first statement should be sent within 30 days of completion of treatment. If no response is received, a second one should be sent within 60 days. This statement should contain wording that will remind patients of overdue accounts while providing them with an opportunity to pay without embarrassment. After 90 days, a special statement should be sent that contains stronger wording. At this point a phone call should follow the statement. After accounts have remained uncollected for 90 days, it is less likely that payment will be received and they may have to be referred to a collection agency or small claims court.

Collection Letters

The patient who receives a collection letter knows that the account is overdue and knows why he or she is receiving the letter. All collection letters should be phrased in firm, positive, business-like terms that make every effort to persuade patients to pay their debts, to help them pay, and to enable them to save face while doing so.

Collection Agencies

The dentist will make the final decision about turning cases over to a collection service. Accounts are never turned over for collection without the employer's knowledge and approval.

Unpaid accounts should be referred for collection while there is still hope of settlement—usually no more than three or four months after the end of treatment. The agency should be given all information which may be helpful and should be kept informed of any new information. The agency should also be notified promptly if the patient pays directly to the dental office.

The collection agency will receive from the patient only the fee due for dental services; no charge for their costs will be added. However, before the collection is remitted to the office, the agency will deduct a

EXHIBIT 11.5 **ACCOUNT STATEMENT**

Fairview Centre Dental Office
3310 Fairview Road
Burlington, Ontario
L7M 3M6

(905)333-3200

ACCOUNT STATEMENT

Fairview Centre Dental Office

DAYS OWING	CURRENT	30-59	60-89	OVER 90	LAST PAYMENT
	247.80				29/JAN/95

Mr. John Sandelli
969 Warburton
Burlington, Ontario
L7M 8L1

DATE	29/JAN/95
ACCOUNT NO.	10109
PLEASE PAY	147.80
AMOUNT ENCLOSED	

PLEASE RETURN THIS PORTION WITH YOUR PAYMENT

RETAIN THIS PORTION FOR YOUR RECORDS

PAGE: 1   ACCOUNT NO.: 10109   AS OF: 29/JAN/95   BALANCE FORWARD: 106.00

DATE	PATIENT	DESCRIPTION	CHARGE	PAYMENT	INS.	BALANCE
29/JAN/95	John	Three Surface Restoration	89.00		31.20	163.80
		Complete Oral Exam	40.00		40.00	163.80
		Two Radiographs	18.00		18.00	163.80
		Porcelain Fused to Metal Crown	475.00		285.00	353.80
29/JAN/95	John	Paid in Cash - Thank You		100.00		253.80
02/FEB/95	Travis	Post-dated Cheque on file Entered: 28/DEC/94		106.00		

John is due after 29/JUL/95 for his 6 month visit.
Ryan has an appointment at 9:00am on Wed 26/APR/95.
Claris has an appointment at 8:50am on Wed 26/APR/95.
Travis has an appointment at 1:10pm on Sat 11/JAN/95.

Clean teeth mean better health.   2% service charge on overdue accounts.
Have a great day!

	CURRENT	30-59	60-89	OVER 90	TOTAL	**PLEASE PAY**
ACCOUNT	247.80	6.00			253.80	147.80
INSURANCE	374.20				374.20	
				TOTAL OBLIGATION	628.00	

Sample provided by ABEL Computers Ltd., Burlington, Ontario.

EXHIBIT 11.6 FIRST COLLECTION LETTER (30 DAYS+ OVERDUE)

Dr. D. Kay
12 Incisor Street, Your City, Province, Postal Code

Date

Mr. Don Smith
123 Any Street
Your City, Province
Postal Code

Dear Mr. Smith:

This is just a friendly reminder of your account balance in the amount of $——. If payment has been forwarded, please disregard this letter. Should you require any further assistance or information, please do not hesitate to contact our office. Thank you.
Sincerely,

Debbi Jones
Office Manager

EXHIBIT 11.6 (cont'd) SECOND COLLECTION LETTER (45–60 DAYS OVERDUE)

Dr. D. Kay
12 Incisor Street, Your City, Province, Postal Code

Date

Mr. Don Smith
123 Any Street
Your City, Province
Postal Code

Dear Mr. Smith:

This letter is to remind you of your account balance in the amount of $——. If you have a question regarding your insurance or if we can be of assistance in helping you make financial arrangements, please do not hesitate to contact our office. Your prompt attention to this matter will be appreciated. Thank you.
Sincerely,

Debbi Jones
Office Manager

EXHIBIT 11.6 (cont'd) **THIRD COLLECTION LETTER (90 DAYS)**

Dr. D. Kay
12 Incisor Street, Your City, Province, Postal Code

Date

Mr. Don Smith
123 Any Street
Your City, Province
Postal Code

Dear Mr. Smith:

We still have not heard from you regarding your account balance in the amount of $———. Every attempt has been made to contact you and to offer our assistance in resolving this problem.

We would like to maintain a good business relationship with you. Therefore, if we can be of assistance in helping you make financial arrangements, please contact our office immediately.

May we please hear from you by _____. At that time it will be necessary to forward your account to a collection service.

Your prompt attention to this matter is essential.

Sincerely,

Debbi Jones
Office Manager

fixed percentage of the total amount collected. Generally, the smaller the amount collected from the patient, the greater the percentage deducted as the collector's fee. For example, a $20 collection might have $10 (50 percent) deducted for costs, but a $300 collection might have only $75 (25 percent) charged against it. Usually, the agency will report results once a month and send a cheque for the net amount due to the dentist.

ASSIGNMENT

1. Define the difference between accounts receivable and accounts payable.
2. In the One Write bookkeeping system, what information is recorded on the records?
3. What information does the patient ledger card show?
4. When is proof of posting done? Why is it done?
5. What factors are taken into consideration when making financial arrangements?
6. What information is necessary to make a financial arrangement with the patient?
7. Calculate the following bookkeeping entries:
   Opening A/R balance is $35,500.00
   a. Mr. Fred Flintstone had restorative work that amounted to $500.00. Fred had a previous balance of $150.00, and he is leaving a cheque today for $350.00. Calculate the current balance.
   b. Mrs. Wilma Waterford had a previous balance of $150.00. She paid Dr. Kay $75.00 cash. Calculate the current balance.
   c. David Todoroff is a transient patient. He had $92.95 worth of restorative work done today. He paid the full amount in cash.
   d. Aynsley Dansk had restorative work done today amounting to $125.00. She paid $120.00 by cheque and her previous balance was $10.00.
   e. Mrs. Tweedledum had a previous balance of $100.00. The dentist asked you to give her a courtesy discount of 10 percent.
   f. You received the following cheques in the mail:
   Jimmy Oliver $40.00—this fully paid his account
   Craig Tuttle $100.00—this paid half of his account
   Balance the daysheet.
8. What is the new accounts receivable balance forward?

CHAPTER TWELVE

ACCOUNTS PAYABLE

OBJECTIVE

At the end of this chapter, the student will be able to identify and describe the following: how to establish a monthly disbursements journal and a method of time management for accounts payable, how to record invoices, packing slips, and statements, how to maintain a continuous bank balance, control costs and redundant ordering through effective inventory control, deal with salespeople, and cross balance the disbursements journal.

TOPICS

- expense categories
- expense records
- verification of invoices/statements/packing slips
- cost control through inventory control
- cross balancing the disbursements journal
- continuous bank balance
- petty cash fund

KEY CONCEPTS

The effective management of a dental office requires organized handling and prompt payment of all bills for practice-related expenses. Because of the complexity of accounting procedures involved, it is important for the dental office administrator to be knowledgeable about single entry bookkeeping and related tasks such as writing cheques, making bank deposits, and maintaining petty cash records.

Most major expense payments are handled by writing a cheque and posting the entry to the appropriate expense category in the disbursements journal. It is helpful for the dental office administrator to be familiar with the business expense categories that are relevant to the individual office. This understanding, along with the proper administrative procedures, can save unnecessary accounting fees and ensure that all records are maintained accurately.

The disbursements journal is a record of all financial transactions made to maintain the office, and its equipment and supplies, as well as employee salary expenses. A continuous bank balance should be maintained to provide the dentist and the accounting service with a "photograph" of the financial status at a given point in time and to ensure that funds are available before cheques are issued. All bills should be approved for payment by the dentist.

THE DISBURSEMENTS JOURNAL

Accounts payable refers to money owed by the practice, and disbursements are the payments of money owed. The disbursements journal should include a record of all deposits and bank charges as well as the cheques that are written. It is usually kept by calendar month.

Each column of the journal breaks down the expenses into the appropriate categories. It is helpful to label each column with the expense category before beginning the monthly disbursements. Keeping the expense categories in the same order from month to month will help to reduce errors.

At the end of each month, the disbursements journal should be cross balanced and the balance carried forward to the next month. The bank balance in the journal should be checked with the true bank balance to ensure that there are sufficient funds in the account and that all transactions have been recorded.

Cross balancing the disbursements journal consists of the following steps:
1. Add up each expense column.
2. Add up the total cheques in the cheque column.
3. The total of the expense columns should equal the total of the cheques column.

EXPENSE CATEGORIES

Expenditures are commonly classified for ease of organization. Classifying expenses into categories helps the accounting service identify the tax deductible expenses. The category headings are used on file folders to store the expense records. At the end of the year, the expense documentation is removed and filed, in the same categories, with other business records for that year.

As each expense cheque is written, it should be subtracted from the continuous bank balance and simultaneously recorded in the appropriate expense category. This will save time allocating expenses.

There are two main types of expenses:

1. *Fixed expenses* include those business expenses that continue at all times. These are costs, such as rent, utilities, and salaries, that go on whether or not the dentist is in the office and whether or not professional services are actually being provided.
2. *Variable expenses* are those, such as supplies, laboratory fees, and repairs, that change depending upon the type of services rendered and the amount consumed.

Description of Expense Categories

1. **Drawings** Lump sum amounts can be transferred to the dentist's personal account to pay personal expenses. It is recommended that only business expenses be paid through the business account. The drawings column will include any personal expenses such as personal insurance, disability and income protection insurance, donations to registered charities, and the practitioner's own personal income tax payments or instalments. Drawings are considered a variable expense.
2. **Salaries and Receiver General Remittances** The net amount of salary cheques as well as the monthly cheque to the Receiver General for employee deductions should be recorded in this expense column. Although there may be some fluctuations, this category is considered to be a fixed expense.
3. **Laboratory Fees** Any fees paid to outside laboratories should be recorded in this column. This information can provide the dentist with a valuable indicator of the practice growth. Laboratory fees are a variable expense.
4. **Professional Supplies** Disbursements for medications, small instruments (usually under $200) and other professional supplies, including patient education pamphlets, tapes, cassettes, etc. are listed here. Due to the unpredictable nature of this expense, it is considered to be variable.

5. **Rent** This is always considered to be a fixed expense when the dentist rents or leases the office premises. This category can also be called "Leasehold."

6. **Office Expenses** General office supplies such as stationery, account cards, appointment books, envelopes, petty cash, waiting room subscriptions, etc. are office expenses. This category is somewhat more predictable in nature but is considered to be a variable expense.

7. **Promotion** Payments of any kind to promote the services of the practice would include club memberships, flowers for patients, donations to unregistered groups, and entertaining bills. This is a variable expense.

8. **Interest and Bank Charges** All bank charges for loan interest, overdraft interest, and service charges are listed here. These charges change from month to month and thus are a variable expense. Bank loan payments generally remain the same each month and should be recorded in a separate column.

9. **Dues and Fees** Any association or membership fees necessary for the maintenance of a professional office are itemized. These fees are usually paid once per year and are considered a fixed expense.

10. **Heat, Hydro, and Water** Payments for heat, light, or water, if paid separately from the rent, are listed in this column. These expenses are fixed, although they may vary slightly from month to month depending on usage.

11. **Insurance** Payments for malpractice, office overhead, and office contents insurance are tax deductible and should be recorded in this column. Please note that the dentist's personal disability, income protection, and life insurance are not tax deductible and should be recorded in "Drawings."

12. **Repairs and Maintenance** General cleaning supplies, janitorial services, and repairs to premises or equipment, etc. are listed in this category.

13. **Telephone** Telephone-related expenses would include costs for regular monthly business service, answering service, etc. This is considered to be a fixed expense.

14. **Bank Loan** Payments on business bank loans are placed in this column. Interest payments should go in the "Interest and Bank Charges" column.

15. **Returned Cheques and Refunds** Returned cheques and refunds to patients may be grouped together and recorded in this column.

16. **Reference Material** Reference materials are professional books or magazines for use by the dentist only. Reception area subscriptions should be classified as an office expense.

17. **Laundry and Uniforms** This category covers amounts paid for the laundering of towels and uniforms. If the dentist provides a uniform allowance as an employment benefit, the cost should be recorded in this column.

18. **Equipment** Any item of office equipment over $100 and any professional instruments costing over $200 should be classified as equipment. A note should indicate what the purchased equipment is. This column will be a variable expense. Because equipment can be depreciated over time, it must be listed separately in this column.

19. **Leasehold Improvements** This column is relevant when outfitting a new office or renovating an old one. Any improvements to rented premises of a lasting nature such as carpentry, electrical installation, painting, wallpapering, carpeting, cabinets, or shelves, which are not removable, fall into this category.

20. **Conventions and Seminars** Use this column for registration fees and expenses incurred for conventions and seminars, including transportation, meals, and accommodations.

21. **Miscellaneous Items** Use this column for expenses for which there is no special column, such as accounting fees, business taxes, or collection fees. A description of the expense should be included. If you are uncertain where to record an expense, put it in "Miscellaneous" with a description and the accounting service will redesignate it later.

WRITING CHEQUES

The basic components of a cheque are

- payee—to whom the cheque is being paid
- payer—whose account the funds are coming out of
- endorsement—signature of the payer
- body and figures—amount of the cheque in numerals (figures) and the amount written out in words
- date—the date the cheque is issued

When writing a cheque, you must be sure that the date is correct, the body and figures agree, and the dentist signs it. One of the most

EXHIBIT 12.1 DISBURSEMENT JOURNAL

DATE	CHEQUE NO.	NAME	EARNINGS REGULAR / OTHER	DEDUCTIONS	CHEQUE AMOUNT	MEMO BALANCE	DEPOSITS DATE	DEPOSITS AMOUNT	DRAWINGS	SALARIES SEC. GEN.	LAB	PROF. SUPPLIES	RENT	OFFICE EXPENSES	PROMOTION DEN CLB.	DUES / FEES	AUTO / HYDRO	INSURANCE
		BALANCES FORWARDED				10,875.09 / 9,875.09												
Jan 2		Drawings to Dr's acct.			1,000 —	9,875.09			1,000 —									
Jan 3	101	Susan Torres - Payroll	1000 —	320.5 4%h 27 wks	647.09	9,226?				647.09								
Jan 4	102	Abby's Lab			540 —	8,687?					540 —							
Jan 4	103	Blue Devies Pharmacy			96.89	8,559.61						96.39						
Jan 4	104	Rent			1,000 —	7,559.61							1,000 —					
Jan ?		Deposit				19,255.39												
Jan 5	105	Filing Direct			67.85	12,375								67.85				
Jan 6	106	Rosengart's Furnishing			55 —	12,324.15								55 —				
Jan 7	107	Public Utility Co.			232 —	12,087.15											232 —	
Jan 7		Deposit				18,5...												
Jan 8	108	Bell Canada			153 —	17,189.15											237 —	
					152.?	17,036.15												
		TOTALS ➝	3,205		3,98.33				1,000 —	647.09	540 —	96.39	1,000 —	67.85 / 55 —			232 — / 237 —	

Used with permission by Safeguard Business Systems, Inc., Fort Washington, PA 19034

EXHIBIT 12.2 **SAMPLE CHEQUE**

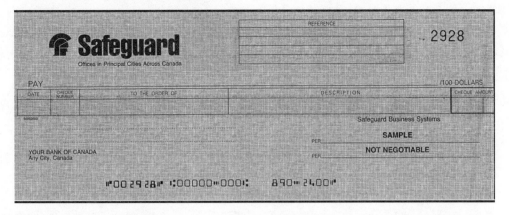

Used with permission by Safeguard Business Systems, Inc., Fort Washington, PA 19034

common errors that occurs in the cheque writing process is using an improper date.

Many business cheques will display a blank block or section on the cheque to record the specific invoice number that the cheque is covering. This block may appear on the cheque stub as well.

A continuous bank balance must be kept in the cheque ledger (stub) of the chequebook. This ensures that there are sufficient funds available for each cheque issued.

It may be helpful to make up a small diary card that identifies when automatic debits or specific payments will be taken from the business account automatically. File the diary card in a chronological file and record the payment on the day that it is due. Automatic bank debits must be recorded to maintain an accurate picture of the bank balance at all times.

If an error should occur when writing the cheque, the word *void* should be written through the cheque. An explanation should be written on the cheque stub and a new cheque issued.

The Petty Cash Fund

Minor expenses are handled through the petty cash fund, which is kept to meet frequent small expenses for which cash is required. The amount in the fund should be large enough to last approximately one month, yet not large enough to invite theft. It should be kept in a locked cabinet or drawer at all times. When the petty cash fund is depleted, it is replenished by writing a cheque.

A petty cash voucher must be submitted for all payments made from the fund. Each voucher must include the date, the amount spent, to whom it was paid, and the reason for the expense. A receipt should be attached to each voucher. Receipts should be kept for all transactions and stapled to a copy of the monthly petty cash fund cheque. The dental office administrator should take responsibility for the petty cash fund and not allow access by others unless a receipt is given.

You can record petty cash transactions in a multicolumn book, or simply use a notebook and draw in three columns on the right-hand side.

When charges or withdrawals are made from the petty cash fund, they are recorded in the debit column. A debit is a charge to an account. When the fund is replenished, the entry will be recorded in the credit column. A credit is a payment to an account.

The petty cash fund should be balanced and replenished on a regular basis, usually once a month. Since there is a voucher for each payment, the sum of all the vouchers plus the cash on hand should always equal the total amount of the petty cash fund. When these have been balanced, a cheque is written to refill the fund. The vouchers and attached receipts are stapled together and dated and the total noted, then they are filed as an office expense.

TABLE 12.1 PETTY CASH FUND RECORDS

BEGIN WITH AN OPENING BALANCE OF $50.00:		Debit	Credit	Balance
Sep. 12	Chq. #177			$50.00
Sep. 19	paperclips	$2.39		47.61
Sep. 20	postage	.78		46.83
Sep. 21	coffee	4.99		41.84
Sep. 25	pens	6.55		35.29
Sep. 30	courier charges	22.05		13.24
Oct. 1	Chq. #235		36.76	50.00

BILL PAYMENTS

Some dentists prefer for the office administrator to pay the bills as they are incurred; others prefer to wait until the supplier's statement is received. Accuracy is essential, so the administrator should try to select a time that is quiet with few distractions.

As invoices and bills are received, they are filed in a subject filing system which will identify each expense by its category. For example, laboratory invoices will be kept in one file and equipment expenses will be kept in another. Invoices will list the charges, but may not itemize the goods received. Often the goods are itemized to help verify that they were received as ordered. A packing slip has a similar purpose but does not usually include the charges.

Statements list all purchases and payments in a given time period, itemizing supplies received and including corresponding invoice numbers.

Before writing cheques to pay the accounts, the dental office administrator should verify all amounts payable by checking the quantities and charges on the invoices received from each supplier during that period against the monthly statement.

The administrator will also check to see that all payments, credits, and returns have been properly entered. To facilitate the handling and storage of records, invoices are stapled to the statement covering them.

INVENTORY CONTROL

Accurate inventory control is essential to good management of office expenses. The control system should be simple and maintained at all times. A clinical staff member could be assigned responsibility for the clinical supplies and the office administrator should take care of stationery, insurance forms, and all of the supplies required for the administration of the office. Carefully monitoring usage of each item is helpful, and knowing the length of time required for reordering and delivery is also important. Identifying the reorder point and flagging it with a reminder sticker or tag will ensure that enough time is allowed.

Effective inventory control will simplify ordering and help to keep operating costs down. Expiry dates on products should be checked and stock should be rotated regularly. Unnecessary ordering along with misuse of supplies will reduce the profit margin of the office.

EXHIBIT 12.3 **SAMPLE REORDER TAG**

Time to Reorder

Product

_____

Supplier

_____

Cost _____

Expected Delivery Date

_____

Ordered by _____

ASSIGNMENT

Set up a disbursements journal with the month and the opening balance. The balance from your previous journal is $10,575.20.

   Pay the following bills:

   a. The first item is an invoice from Standard Dental Supplies for $108.00. Pay this bill using cheque #1

   b. Cheque #2 is to be written to D & L Labs for $263.00

   c. Cheque #3 is to be written to City Hydro Electric for $271.25

   Record the following transactions:

   d. You made a deposit today in the amount of $4,000.00

   e. You wrote a payroll cheque to Janice Green for $573.50.

   f. You paid the cleaning staff $85.00.

   Please cross balance your journal. What is your journal balance forward?

   _____

CHAPTER THIRTEEN

PAYROLL

OBJECTIVE

At the end of this chapter, the student will be able to identify and describe the following: an employee payroll record, a Record of Employment, and a T4 slip, payroll records for new employees, the monthly remittance to Revenue Canada, and the PD7A form. The student will also understand the procedures for termination of staff.

TOPICS

- time records
- new employees
- the TD1 form
- source deductions
- unemployment insurance
- Canada Pension Plan
- income tax
- deduction/remittance
- T4 Summary of Remuneration

PAYROLL CONSIDERATIONS

Dentists may employ an accounting or payroll service to administer the staff payroll. In most offices, however, the dental office administrator is the person responsible for the appropriate and accurate administration of staff remuneration. It is essential to maintain accurate and complete records of the hours worked, deductions, and government remittances. It is equally important to protect the confidential nature of the records. The administrator should not discuss salaries with staff members, particularly in an open area where patients or other staff members can hear. Salary negotiations should occur privately between the dentist and each individual staff member. The office administrator would be committing a breach of trust by releasing confidential information.

Payroll and source deduction information is readily available from Revenue Canada, Source Deductions Department. In many cities, local offices offer free seminars for small business payroll administrators. If the seminars are not available, you may be able to obtain a complete kit of source deduction information for small businesses. Do not hesitate to call the local Source Deductions office when questions arise concerning employee deductions. If deductions are withheld and submitted incorrectly, the dental office could face penalties.

Payroll records should be retained for a minimum of six years. Most offices, however, will retain records indefinitely. The records should be kept locked in a fireproof cabinet or safe.

Time Records

Time records should be kept for all part-time, hourly, and salaried employees. These include regular, overtime, and vacation hours, as well as weekend shifts and holidays. A payroll journal can be obtained from any office supply store. It is also helpful to use the payroll journal information provided on the One Write system available through Safeguard Business Systems.

NEW EMPLOYEES

When an employee is hired, the following information must be obtained:
- employee's full legal name, including middle initial
- social insurance number
- complete address of the employee, including postal code
- date hired
- appropriate tax claim code, which is obtained from the TD1 form
- hourly rate, if applicable

Every new employee should fill out a TD1 form to determine the proper claim code. The TD1, shown partially on page 154 as Exhibit 13.2, is a tax form that determines what the employee's basic personal

EXHIBIT 13.1   **PAYROLL RECORD FORM**

PAYROLL RECORD

Name   S.I.N.

Date Hired

Address   Postal code

D.O.B.

GROSS PAY	INSURABLE EARNINGS	INCOME TAX	EI	CPP	TOTAL DEDUCTIONS	NET PAY

tax exemption will be. This ensures that the correct amount of income tax is deducted at each pay period.

An employee who wants additional tax taken from his or her pay each week must complete a new TD1. Line 18 of this form must be completed specifying how much additional tax should be taken. Additional tax can be taken off in increments of $5, $10, $15, $20, etc. The TD1 form should be retained with the employee's payroll record and updated periodically, perhaps once a year, to ensure that the information is current.

If an employee does not complete a TD1 form, the payroll administrator should use claim code 1 and deduct income tax as if the employee is single. If the employee is a nonresident, claim code 0 should be used.

Social Insurance Number

The social insurance number (SIN) is used to identify Canada Pension Plan contributions as well as employment insurance claims. It is most important that a new employee's correct social insurance number is provided at the start of employment. Using the wrong number could cause considerable delay or reduce the employee's entitlement to benefits in the future. Employers are responsible for ensuring that all employees who do not have a social insurance number apply to obtain one.

EXHIBIT 13.2 PERSONAL TAX CREDITS RETURN

Revenue   Revenu
Canada   Canada

PERSONAL TAX CREDITS RETURN

After you complete this return, give it to your employer or payer.

Last name (capital letters)	Usual first name and initials	Employee number

Address	For non-residents only - country of permanent residence	Social insurance number

	Postal code		Date of birth
			Year Month Day

1. Basic personal amount

Everyone can claim **$6,456** as the basic personal amount.
- If you choose to claim this amount, **enter $ 6,456** .
- If you choose not to claim this amount (e.g. , when you have more than one employer or payer and you have already claimed the basic personal amount), **enter 0** in box **A** on the other side of this return and do not complete sections 2 to 8. You may wish to complete sections 9 to 11.
- If you are a non-resident, and you will be including most of your annual world income (90% or more) when determining your taxable income in Canada, you can claim certain personal amounts. If you are not sure about your non-resident status, or need more information, call the Client Assistance Division of your income tax office.   **Credit claimed $**

2. Spousal amount or equivalent-to-spouse amount.

You can claim an amount for supporting your spouse if you are **married or have a common-law spouse**. A common-law spouse is a person of the opposite sex with whom you live in a common-law relationship for any continuous period of at least 12 months, including any period of separation (due to a breakdown in the relationship) of less than 90 days, or with whom you live in a common-law relationship and who is the natural or adoptive parent of your child.

You can claim an equivalent-to-spouse amount if you are **single, divorced, separated, or widowed,** and you support a relative who is:
- residing in Canada (if the relative is your child, the child does not have to reside in Canada);
- living with you in a home you maintain;
- related to you by blood, marriage, or adoption; and
- under 18 years old, except for a relative who has a mental or physical infirmity.

Calculating the amount

If you marry during the year, your spouse's net income includes the income earned before and during the marriage.
If the net income of your spouse or relative for the year will be:
- over $5,918, **enter 0**;
- $538 or less, **enter $5,380**; or
- more than $538, complete calculation no. 2 on the back of this return and enter the result as credit claimed.

                                                                          Credit claimed $
Any person you claim here cannot be claimed again in section 3.

3. Amount for disabled dependent relatives

With the introduction of the child tax benefit, there is no amount for dependent children who are under the age of 18 at the end of the year. However, you can claim an amount for each disabled dependant who is:
- your or your spouse's child or grandchild, 18 years old or older, and who has a physical or mental infirmity; or
- your or your spouse's parent, grandparent, brother, sister, aunt, uncle, niece, or nephew, who is 18 years old or older, and who has a physical or mental infirmity and is resident in Canada.

Calculating the amount for a disabled dependent relative:

If your dependant's net income for the year will be:
- $2,690 or less, **enter $1,583** in section 3 of this return; or
- more than $2,690, complete calculation no. 3 on the back of this return and enter the result as credit claimed.
You can claim an amount for each disabled dependent relative you have.   **Credit claimed $**

4. Amount for eligible pension

An eligible pension income includes pension payments received from a pension plan or fund as a life annuity, and foreign pension payments. It does not include payments from the Canada or Quebec Pension Plan, Old Age Security, guaranteed supplements, or lump-sum withdrawals from a pension fund.

If you receive an eligible pension income, you can claim your eligible pension income or
$1,000, whichever amount is less.   **Credit claimed $**

5. Age amount .

If your estimated net income from all sources for the year will be:
- $ 25,921 or less, **enter $3,482** ;
- over $25,921, but not over $49,134.33, complete calculation no. 5 on the back of this return and **enter** the result as credit claimed; or
- over $49,134.33, **enter $0**.   **Credit claimed $**

Reproduced with the permission of Revenue Canada and the Minister of Public Works and Government Services Canada, 1996.

The first digit of the social insurance number indicates the region of the country where the card was issued. Foreign citizens or landed immigrants will have a SIN beginning with 9, and they must have a temporary work permit which states they will be working for that employer only. Hiring a person who does not have a work permit is an offence under the Canada Immigration Act which may subject the dentist to risk of penalty.

THE EMPLOYER/EMPLOYEE RELATIONSHIP

The first step in payroll administration is to determine if an employer/employee relationship exists. In most cases, there will be no difficulty in determining whether someone is an employee. If doubt exists, however, a specific ruling should be obtained from the district Revenue Canada office. A form, CPT1 *Request for a Ruling as to the Status of a Worker under the Canada Pension Plan or Unemployment Insurance Act,* is available for this purpose.

Why is this relevant to the dental office administrator?

A dental hygienist or other personnel may ask to be paid as a private contractor. Private contractors are responsible for submitting their own deductions to Revenue Canada; therefore, it is not necessary to withhold deductions at the source. As a payroll administrator, you must comply with the rules and regulations that are applicable to the situation. Failure to submit the necessary source deductions to Revenue Canada can result in the employer being liable for the full amount of the employee's contributions and premiums, plus the employer's contributions and premiums on behalf of the employee. In addition, the employer will be subject to any applicable penalties. In order to protect the employer from unnecessary penalties, you should obtain the special ruling from the employee who wishes to work as a subcontractor and retain this with the payroll records. If the employee fails to produce the special ruling, withhold and submit the appropriate deductions as usual.

SOURCE DEDUCTIONS

Source deductions are subtracted from the gross earnings of every employee. The gross pay is the rate of pay before deductions are withheld. The pay that remains after deductions is called the net pay.

All employers must withhold the following deductions:

- income tax
- Canada Pension Plan contribution (CPP)
- Employment insurance (EI) premiums.

Deductions should be taken according to the rules and regulations stated in the *Employer's Guide to Payroll Deductions,* available from Revenue Canada.

Income Tax

New Tax Deductions Tables are sent to each employer by January 1 each year. (See Exhibit 13.3.)

To use the table, the dental office administrator finds the total amount of gross earnings in the left column under the appropriate pay period. Under the column that contains the tax claim code (at the top of the page), the correct amount of income tax to be deducted is shown. The employer submits the exact amount of income tax that is deducted from the employee's gross earnings to Revenue Canada.

Canada Pension Plan

A Canada Pension Plan deduction is taken from all earnings, provided that the employee is over 18 years of age and under 70 years of age, up to an annual maximum specified in the *Payroll Deduction Tables* from Revenue Canada. The maximum contribution is usually reached some time in November, if the employee has worked for a full year. If the CPP deduction is taken above the maximum, the employee will be refunded the additional amount when he or she submits an income tax return. If the employee changes jobs and has already reached the annual maximum CPP contribution, the new employer takes deductions as if no others have been taken.

The employer is responsible for submitting 100 percent of the employee's contribution. In other words, the total CPP contribution that is submitted to Revenue Canada will be the amount that is withheld from the employee's pay along with a matched contribution from the employer.

Employment Insurance

It is important for the dental office administrator to be aware of the rules and regulations regarding the insurability of earnings. The

EXHIBIT 13.3 TAX DEDUCTIONS TABLES

Canada Pension Plan Contributions Biweekly (26 pay periods a year)					Cotisations au Régime de pensions du Canada Aux deux semaines (26 périodes de paie par année)			

Pay Rémunération		CPP RPC	Pay Rémunération		CPP RPC	Pay Rémunération		CPP RPC	Pay Rémunération		CPP RPC
From - De	To - À		From - De	To - À		From - De	To - À		From - De	To - À	
545.86 -	546.21	11.52	571.58 -	571.93	12.24	597.29 -	597.64	12.96	623.01 -	623.35	13.68
546.22 -	546.57	11.53	571.94 -	572.28	12.25	597.65 -	598.00	12.97	623.36 -	623.71	13.69
546.58 -	546.93	11.54	572.29 -	572.64	12.26	598.01 -	598.35	12.98	623.72 -	624.07	13.70
546.94 -	547.28	11.55	572.65 -	573.00	12.27	598.36 -	598.71	12.99	624.08 -	624.43	13.71
547.29 -	547.64	11.56	573.01 -	573.35	12.28	598.72 -	599.07	13.00	624.44 -	624.78	13.72
547.65 -	548.00	11.57	573.36 -	573.71	12.29	599.08 -	599.43	13.01	624.79 -	625.14	13.73
548.01 -	548.35	11.58	573.72 -	574.07	12.30	599.44 -	599.78	13.02	625.15 -	625.50	13.74
548.36 -	548.71	11.59	574.08 -	574.43	12.31	599.79 -	600.14	13.03	625.51 -	625.85	13.75
548.72 -	549.07	11.60	574.44 -	574.78	12.32	600.15 -	600.50	13.04	625.86 -	626.21	13.76
549.08 -	549.43	11.61	574.79 -	575.14	12.33	600.51 -	600.85	13.05	626.22 -	626.57	13.77
549.44 -	549.78	11.62	575.15 -	575.50	12.34	600.86 -	601.21	13.06	626.58 -	626.93	13.78
549.79 -	550.14	11.63	575.51 -	575.85	12.35	601.22 -	601.57	13.07	626.94 -	627.28	13.79
550.15 -	550.50	11.64	575.86 -	576.21	12.36	601.58 -	601.93	13.08	627.29 -	627.64	13.80
550.51 -	550.85	11.65	576.22 -	576.57	12.37	601.94 -	602.28	13.09	627.65 -	628.00	13.81
550.86 -	551.21	11.66	576.58 -	576.93	12.38	602.29 -	602.64	13.10	628.01 -	628.35	13.82
551.22 -	551.57	11.67	576.94 -	577.28	12.39	602.65 -	603.00	13.11	628.36 -	628.71	13.83
551.58 -	551.93	11.68	577.29 -	577.64	12.40	603.01 -	603.35	13.12	628.72 -	629.07	13.84
551.94 -	552.28	11.69	577.65 -	578.00	12.41	603.36 -	603.71	13.13	629.08 -	629.43	13.85
552.29 -	552.64	11.70	578.01 -	578.35	12.42	603.72 -	604.07	13.14	629.44 -	629.78	13.86
552.65 -	553.00	11.71	578.36 -	578.71	12.43	604.08 -	604.43	13.15	629.79 -	630.14	13.87
553.01 -	553.35	11.72	578.72 -	579.07	12.44	604.44 -	604.78	13.16	630.15 -	630.50	13.88
553.36 -	553.71	11.73	579.08 -	579.43	12.45	604.79 -	605.14	13.17	630.51 -	630.85	13.89
553.72 -	554.07	11.74	579.44 -	579.78	12.46	605.15 -	605.50	13.18	630.86 -	631.21	13.90
554.08 -	554.43	11.75	579.79 -	580.14	12.47	605.51 -	605.85	13.19	631.22 -	631.57	13.91
554.44 -	554.78	11.76	580.15 -	580.50	12.48	605.86 -	606.21	13.20	631.58 -	631.93	13.92
554.79 -	555.14	11.77	580.51 -	580.85	12.49	606.22 -	606.57	13.21	631.94 -	632.28	13.93
555.15 -	555.50	11.78	580.86 -	581.21	12.50	606.58 -	606.93	13.22	632.29 -	632.64	13.94
555.51 -	555.85	11.79	581.22 -	581.57	12.51	606.94 -	607.28	13.23	632.65 -	633.00	13.95
555.86 -	556.21	11.80	581.58 -	581.93	12.52	607.29 -	607.64	13.24	633.01 -	633.35	13.96
556.22 -	556.57	11.81	581.94 -	582.28	12.53	607.65 -	608.00	13.25	633.36 -	633.71	13.97
556.58 -	556.93	11.82	582.29 -	582.64	12.54	608.01 -	608.35	13.26	633.72 -	634.07	13.98
556.94 -	557.28	11.83	582.65 -	583.00	12.55	608.36 -	608.71	13.27	634.08 -	634.43	13.99
557.29 -	557.64	11.84	583.01 -	583.35	12.56	608.72 -	609.07	13.28	634.44 -	634.78	14.00
557.65 -	558.00	11.85	583.36 -	583.71	12.57	609.08 -	609.43	13.29	634.79 -	635.14	14.01
558.01 -	558.35	11.86	583.72 -	584.07	12.58	609.44 -	609.78	13.30	635.15 -	635.50	14.02
558.36 -	558.71	11.87	584.08 -	584.43	12.59	609.79 -	610.14	13.31	635.51 -	635.85	14.03
558.72 -	559.07	11.88	584.44 -	584.78	12.60	610.15 -	610.50	13.32	635.86 -	636.21	14.04
559.08 -	559.43	11.89	584.79 -	585.14	12.61	610.51 -	610.85	13.33	636.22 -	636.57	14.05
559.44 -	559.78	11.90	585.15 -	585.50	12.62	610.86 -	611.21	13.34	636.58 -	636.93	14.06
559.79 -	560.14	11.91	585.51 -	585.85	12.63	611.22 -	611.57	13.35	636.94 -	637.28	14.07
560.15 -	560.50	11.92	585.86 -	586.21	12.64	611.58 -	611.93	13.36	637.29 -	637.64	14.08
560.51 -	560.85	11.93	586.22 -	586.57	12.65	611.94 -	612.28	13.37	637.65 -	638.00	14.09
560.86 -	561.21	11.94	586.58 -	586.93	12.66	612.29 -	612.64	13.38	638.01 -	638.35	14.10
561.22 -	561.57	11.95	586.94 -	587.28	12.67	612.65 -	613.00	13.39	638.36 -	638.71	14.11
561.58 -	561.93	11.96	587.29 -	587.64	12.68	613.01 -	613.35	13.40	638.72 -	639.07	14.12
561.94 -	562.28	11.97	587.65 -	588.00	12.69	613.36 -	613.71	13.41	639.08 -	639.43	14.13
562.29 -	562.64	11.98	588.01 -	588.35	12.70	613.72 -	614.07	13.42	639.44 -	639.78	14.14
562.65 -	563.00	11.99	588.36 -	588.71	12.71	614.08 -	614.43	13.43	639.79 -	640.14	14.15
563.01 -	563.35	12.00	588.72 -	589.07	12.72	614.44 -	614.78	13.44	640.15 -	640.50	14.16
563.36 -	563.71	12.01	589.08 -	589.43	12.73	614.79 -	615.14	13.45	640.51 -	640.85	14.17
563.72 -	564.07	12.02	589.44 -	589.78	12.74	615.15 -	615.50	13.46	640.86 -	641.21	14.18
564.08 -	564.43	12.03	589.79 -	590.14	12.75	615.51 -	615.85	13.47	641.22 -	641.57	14.19
564.44 -	564.78	12.04	590.15 -	590.50	12.76	615.86 -	616.21	13.48	641.58 -	641.93	14.20
564.79 -	565.14	12.05	590.51 -	590.85	12.77	616.22 -	616.57	13.49	641.94 -	642.28	14.21
565.15 -	565.50	12.06	590.86 -	591.21	12.78	616.58 -	616.93	13.50	642.29 -	642.64	14.22
565.51 -	565.85	12.07	591.22 -	591.57	12.79	616.94 -	617.28	13.51	642.65 -	643.00	14.23
565.86 -	566.21	12.08	591.58 -	591.93	12.80	617.29 -	617.64	13.52	643.01 -	643.35	14.24
566.22 -	566.57	12.09	591.94 -	592.28	12.81	617.65 -	618.00	13.53	643.36 -	643.71	14.25
566.58 -	566.93	12.10	592.29 -	592.64	12.82	618.01 -	618.35	13.54	643.72 -	644.07	14.26
566.94 -	567.28	12.11	592.65 -	593.00	12.83	618.36 -	618.71	13.55	644.08 -	644.43	14.27
567.29 -	567.64	12.12	593.01 -	593.35	12.84	618.72 -	619.07	13.56	644.44 -	644.78	14.28
567.65 -	568.00	12.13	593.36 -	593.71	12.85	619.08 -	619.43	13.57	644.79 -	645.14	14.29
568.01 -	568.35	12.14	593.72 -	594.07	12.86	619.44 -	619.78	13.58	645.15 -	645.50	14.30
568.36 -	568.71	12.15	594.08 -	594.43	12.87	619.79 -	620.14	13.59	645.51 -	645.85	14.31
568.72 -	569.07	12.16	594.44 -	594.78	12.88	620.15 -	620.50	13.60	645.86 -	646.21	14.32
569.08 -	569.43	12.17	594.79 -	595.14	12.89	620.51 -	620.85	13.61	646.22 -	646.57	14.33
569.44 -	569.78	12.18	595.15 -	595.50	12.90	620.86 -	621.21	13.62	646.58 -	646.93	14.34
569.79 -	570.14	12.19	595.51 -	595.85	12.91	621.22 -	621.57	13.63	646.94 -	647.28	14.35
570.15 -	570.50	12.20	595.86 -	596.21	12.92	621.58 -	621.93	13.64	647.29 -	647.64	14.36
570.51 -	570.85	12.21	596.22 -	596.57	12.93	621.94 -	622.28	13.65	647.65 -	648.00	14.37
570.86 -	571.21	12.22	596.58 -	596.93	12.94	622.29 -	622.64	13.66	648.01 -	648.35	14.38
571.22 -	571.57	12.23	596.94 -	597.28	12.95	622.65 -	623.00	13.67	648.36 -	648.71	14.39

Employee's maximum CPP contribution for the year 1996 is $893.20   La cotisation maximale de l'employé au RPC pour l'année 1996 est de 893,20 $

B-12

Reproduced with permission of Revenue Canada and the Minister of Public Works and Government Services Canada, 1996.

TABLE 13.1 CPP CONTRIBUTIONS

Employee CPP contribution +	Employer CPP contribution =	Total CPP contribution
$20.00	$20.00	$40.00

regulations affect the amount of deductions taken from the employee, as well as the employer's contribution. An employer is responsible for submitting 1.4 times the amount of the employee's premiums on insurable earnings for the pay period.

Remitting Deductions

All employee deductions including the employer's portion must be remitted to the Receiver General by the 15th of the subsequent month. For example, the deductions for the month of January will be due on February 15. These can be paid at the bank using the government remittance form called a PD7A.

A fast method of calculating the monthly deductions is shown in Table 13.2.

TABLE 13.2 CALCULATING DEDUCTIONS FOR REMITTANCE

EMPLOYEE	INCOME TAX	CPP	EI
J. Smith	106.30	8.85	8.10
S. Brown	131.06	9.05	9.77
SUBTOTALS	237.36	17.90	17.87
		×2	×2.4
TOTALS	237.36	35.80	42.88

TOTAL REMITTED TO THE RECEIVER GENERAL FOR CANADA

$237.36
+ 35.80
+ 42.88
$316.04

EXHIBIT 13.4 DEDUCTIONS REMITTANCE FORM

Revenue Canada Customs, Excise and Taxation | Revenu Canada Accise, Douanes et Impôt

STATEMENT OF ACCOUNT PD7A(E) Rev.93

1 Account number Employer name

Statement of account as of	Amount paid for	Assessed amount owing	You can make your payment where you bank or to:
			Taxation Centre
Transactions processed after this date will appear on the next statement	For enquiries contact		

• IMPORTANT - SEE REVERSE •

EXPLANATION OF CHANGES

Date	Description	Amount

Indicate remittance information in this area for your records

CPP contributions	UI premiums	Tax deductions	Current payment	Gross monthly payroll	No. of empl. - last period

2 Account number Employer name PD7A(E) Rev.93

PIERRE GRAVELLE, QC
DEPUTY MINISTER, DEPARTMENT OF NATIONAL REVENUE, TAXATION

3 Revenue Canada Customs, Excise and Taxation | Revenu Canada Accise, Douanes et Impôt

REMITTANCE FORM FOR CURRENT SOURCE DEDUCTIONS PD7A(E) Rev.93

6 Account number | For Taxation use only

Amount of payment

Month for which deductions were withheld — Year — Month

Gross monthly payroll (dollars only) 0 0

Number of employees in last pay period

Reproduced with permission of Revenue Canada and the Minister of Public Works and Government Services Canada, 1996.

The exact amount of income tax is remitted as it is deducted. There is no employer contribution required. The employer must match the CPP contributions and pay 1.4 times (or 140 percent) of the amount of the EI deduction.

The PD7A, usually a two- or three-part form, is mailed to the dental office automatically each month. The Employer Number or account number appears on each section of the form. This number identifies the employer to Revenue Canada. There are spaces available to record the details of the remittance (i.e., tax deductions, CPP contributions, and EI premiums) along with the total amount of the remittance. The month in which the deductions were made will be displayed in the third section under "Month for which deductions were withheld."

Parts 1 and 3 of the PD7A form should accompany the payment. Part 1 will be returned to the dental office as a receipt. Part 2 of the PD7A should be retained in the payroll records as a record of payment. If the PD7A form has not been received or if it has been misplaced, a cheque can be sent to the District Taxation Centre giving the employer number and indicating the period covered by the remittance.

The dental office administrator should prepare a diary card as a reminder to remit the deductions on time. Remember that after 3:00 p.m., many banks change their transaction dates to the next day. This may lead to a late payment charge. All parts of the form will be dated with the bank teller's verification stamp.

T4 Slips

Every employer is required to forward completed T4 Supplementary and related T4 Summary forms to the appropriate taxation centre, on or before the last day of February each year for the preceding calendar year. Two copies of Form T4 Supplementary *Statement of Remuneration Paid* must be mailed to the employee's latest known address or delivered to the employee in person on or before the same date. The latter form summarizes the total deductions that were withheld from the employee's pay and is needed to prepare personal tax returns.

VACATION PAY

An employee is entitled to 4 percent of their gross pay annually as vacation pay, following the first full year of employment. This equates to two weeks paid vacation. Vacation pay should be treated as a regular paycheque with the appropriate deductions taken. Indicate paid vacation on the payroll records.

RECORD OF EMPLOYMENT

Every time an employee experiences an interruption of earnings, the employer must issue a *Record of Employment*. This may occur when the employment has ended (i.e., the employee quits or is fired) or the employee leaves because of illness, injury, pregnancy, adoption leave, layoff, or leave without pay.

The *Record of Employment* must be issued within five days of the employer becoming aware there has been an interruption of earnings. *Record of Employment* forms and a complete guide entitled *How to Complete the Record of Employment* may be obtained from the local Canada Employment Centre.

It is important that the *Record of Employment* is completed in a timely and accurate manner, as it contains important information that affects the wage replacement benefit that the employee is entitled to.

The Record of Employment will reflect the last 20 weeks of insurable earnings. This is the amount that payment to the claimant is based on. Maintaining accurate payroll records will make the completion of this form a simple process. If an interruption of earnings occurs, the payroll administrator can simply refer to the payroll records to accurately complete the *Record of Employment*.

To summarize, when an employee quits or is fired,

1. Any outstanding vacation pay must be paid and the appropriate deductions withheld.
2. A *Record of Employment* form should be completed and given to the employee within five days of departure.
3. The current address of the employee should be verified to ensure that the T4 Summary will be received at the end of the year.

For any problems or any questions regarding the administration of payroll, the dental office administrator can refer to *Employers Guide to Payroll Deductions: Basic Information* or the *Payroll Deductions Tables* published by Revenue Canada, or contact the local taxation office.

EXHIBIT 13.5 T4 SUMMARY AND STATEMENT OF REMUNERATION PAID

Revenue Canada / Revenu Canada

T4 SUMMARY SOMMAIRE

0505 44111

1994

Complete this return using the instructions in the *Employers' Guide to Payroll Deductions - Basic Information.*

Vous devez remplir cette déclaration selon les instructions du *Guide de l'employeur – Retenues sur la paie : Renseignements de base.*

SUMMARY OF REMUNERATION PAID
(For the year ending December 31, 1994)

SOMMAIRE DE LA RÉMUNÉRATION PAYÉE
(Pour l'année se terminant le 31 décembre 1994)

Copy / Copie 1

If you file your T4 return on tape or diskette, you no longer need to complete this form. See the guide called *Computer Specifications for Data Filed on Magnetic Media* for more information.

Si vous produisez votre déclaration T4 sur disquette ou sur bande, vous n'avez plus à remplir ce formulaire. Consultez le guide *Spécifications informatiques pour données produites sur support magnétique* pour obtenir plus d'informations.

Important

Employer's name and number must be the same as those shown on your PD7A remittance form. The T4 Summary must be filed on or before February 28, 1995.

Le nom et le numéro de l'employeur doivent être les mêmes que ceux qui figurent sur le formulaire de versement PD7A. La T4 Sommaire doit être produite au plus tard le 28 février 1995.

Account number / Numéro de compte

Name and address of employer / Nom et adresse de l'employeur

Taxation centre / Centre fiscal

DO code / Code du BD

T4 Supplementary slips totals

For returns with over 300 T4 slips, please see instructions in the *Employers' Guide to Payroll Deductions - Basic Information* about the breakdown of large returns.

Totaux des feuillets T4 *Supplémentaire*

Pour les déclarations renfermant plus de 300 feuillets T4, consultez le *Guide de l'employeur – Retenues sur la paie : Renseignements de base* pour la répartition des déclarations volumineuses.

Of the total number at left, indicate how many T4 slips are for employees whose addresses are in the U.S.A.

Indiquez le nombre de feuillets T4 total émis pour des employés dont l'adresse est au É.-U.

Field	Description FR	Box
Total number of T4 slips filed	Nombre total de feuillets T4 produits	88
Employment income before deductions	Revenus d'emploi avant retenues	14
Registered pension plan contributions	Cotisations à un régime de pension agréé	20
Pension adjustment	Facteur d'équivalence	52
Unemployment insurance insurable earnings	Gains assurables d'assurance-chômage	24
Employee's Canada Pension Plan contributions	Cotisations de l'employé au Régime de pensions du Canada	16
Employer's Canada Pension Plan contributions	Cotisations de l'employeur au Régime de pensions du Canada	27
Employee's Unemployment Insurance premiums	Cotisations de l'employé à l'assurance-chômage	18
Employer's Unemployment Insurance premiums	Cotisations de l'employeur à l'assurance-chômage	19
Income tax deducted	Impôt sur le revenu retenu	22

Departmental use only

Total deductions reported (16 + 27 + 18 + 19 + 22) / Total des retenues déclarées (16 + 27 + 18 + 19 + 22) — 80

Minus: remittances – Moins : versements — 82

Difference – Différence

We do not charge or refund a difference of less than $2.00.
Une différence inférieure à 2 $ ne sera ni exigée ni remboursée par le Ministère.

Overpayment / Montant du trop-payé — 84

Balance due / Solde à payer — 86

* If you have not paid the total deductions reported, include the balance with this completed return. You may have to pay a penalty for late payment if you have any balance owing.

Si vous n'avez pas payé le montant total des retenues déclarées, veuillez joindre le solde à payer, à la présente déclaration. Tout solde à payer est assujetti à une pénalité pour paiement tardif.

Amount enclosed / Somme jointe

Revenue Canada issued – registration number(s) for RPP or DPSP – Numéro(s) d'enregistrement émis par Revenu Canada pour le RPA ou le RPDB

71   72   73

Canadian-controlled private corporations or unincorporated employers: list the social insurance number of the main shareholder(s) or proprietor(s).
Sociétés privées dont le contrôle est canadien ou employeurs non constitués: Inscrivez le numéro d'assurance sociale de l'(des) actionnaire(s) ou du (des) propriétaire(s).

74   75

Réservé au Ministère

Person to contact about this return – Personne avec qui communiquer au sujet de cette déclaration — 76

First name – Prénom   Surname – Nom de famille

Telephone number – Numéro de téléphone — 78

Area code – Indicatif régional

Certification – Attestation

I certify that the information given in this T4 return (T4 Summary and related T4 Supplementary slips) is, to the best of my knowledge, correct and complete.

J'atteste que les renseignements fournis dans cette déclaration T4 (la T4 Sommaire et les feuillets T4 Supplémentaire connexes) sont, à ma connaissance, exacts et complets.

Date | Name and surname (in capital letters) – Nom et prénom (en lettres majuscules) | Signature of authorized person – Signature de la personne autorisée | Position or office – Titre ou poste

For departmental use only: please do not write in this area – Réservé au Ministère : Ne rien écrire ici

90	Transfer / Transfert	1	Least to current / Précédente à courante	91	Pro Forma	1	No / Non	93	Date	Memo – Notes
		2	No action / Aucune mesure			2	Yes / Oui	94		A
		3	Other / Autre							B

Late-filing penalty / Pénalité pour production tardive

Prepared by – Établi par   Date

| Initials – Initiales | Code 2 | Correspond. | Inc. | TPC – CCT | Dressed – MAP | Rev. – Rév. | No Accounts – Aucun n° |
| Date | | | | | | | |

* Keep the working copy of this Summary for your records.
* Send copies 1 and 2 of this Summary and copy 1 of the related T4 Supplementary to the appropriate taxation centre address in box A on the back of this form.

* Conservez le brouillon du formulaire T4 Sommaire pour vos dossiers.
* Envoyez les copies 1 et 2 du formulaire T4 Sommaire ainsi que la copie 1 du T4 Supplémentaire connexes au centre fiscal approprié, dont l'adresse figure à la case A au verso de ce formulaire.

Reproduced with permission of Revenue Canada and the Minister of Public Works and Government Services Canada, 1996.

EXHIBIT 13.5 (continued) **T4 SUMMARY AND STATEMENT OF REMUNERATION PAID**

Reproduced with permission of Revenue Canada and the Minister of Public Works and Government Services Canada, 1996.

ASSIGNMENT

1. Obtain *Payroll Deductions Tables* from the local taxation office and complete the payroll record for the following employees (your office is on a biweekly payroll):

   a. Heidi Hygiene worked 80 hours and made $25 per hour. Her tax claim code is 3.

   b. Rita Reception worked 80 hours and made $15 per hour. Her tax claim code is 1.

   c. Penny Partime worked 35 hours at $6 per hour. Her tax claim code is 1.

PAYROLL RECORD

GROSS PAY	INSURABLE EARNINGS	INCOME TAX	EI	CPP	TOTAL DEDUCTIONS	NET PAY

2. Calculate your remittance to the Receiver General.

   Income Tax _____

   CPP _____

   EI _____

   Total Remittance _____

CHAPTER FOURTEEN

BANKING

OBJECTIVE

At the end of this chapter, the student will be able to identify and describe the following: how to maintain current financial records and the importance of accuracy, how to complete a bank deposit slip, balancing the daily bank deposit to the payments made, and reconciling the monthly bank statement.

TOPICS

- bank services
- current accounts
- payment options
- stop payment orders
- bank statements
- reconciliation

RESPONSIBILITIES

One of the daily responsibilities of the dental office administrator is to oversee all payments received and to ensure that they are appropriately deposited, while maintaining a consecutive bank balance. You must understand basic bank services and know how to write cheques, prepare deposit slips, and reconcile the bank statement monthly. In some dental practices, the dentist or his or her spouse may prefer to control the bank account; however, in most circumstances it is one of the many responsibilities of the dental office administrator.

BANK SERVICES

There are numerous banking services that are available to small businesses, such as dental offices, and there is considerable competition between financial institutions to acquire and maintain business accounts. Depending on which financial institution is selected, an account representative may be assigned to handle questions and provide assistance with specific banking needs.

The dental office administrator should be familiar with the type of account dealt with and the regulations and service charges that are applicable.

Current Accounts

Each dental office will have at least one commercial or business chequing account. This type of account is known as a current account. Current accounts are intended to be used for commercial purposes. They are opened in the name of the business, the dentist, or the dental office. Current accounts are handled in a somewhat different manner than personal chequing accounts. A current account may not be overdrawn; however, a line of credit may be established between the dentist and the financial institution. This is also known as revolving credit. Essentially it means that if there are not sufficient funds in the account, funds will be advanced in the form of a loan. The dentist must sign a series of promissory notes when the line of credit is established. As funds are deposited to the account, the loan (or promissory note) is paid.

When a current account is established, the dentist will determine who is to be granted the authority to sign cheques on the commercial account. The bank will require the dentist or principal owners of the practice to complete signing authority documents for this purpose. The dentist may require that the dental office administrator have joint authority to sign on the current accounts, in which case the signatures of both the dentist and the administrator are required on each cheque. In most cases, however, the dentist maintains control of the current account and signs every cheque before it leaves the office.

Cheques

A cheque is a written order in which a bank is required to pay a designated sum to the bearer. Payment is on demand, which means that when the cheque is presented to the bank, that amount of money must be paid, as long as there are sufficient funds in the account to cover the amount of the cheque.

The *payee* is the person named on the cheque as the intended recipient of the amount shown. The name of the designated payee will usually follow the words "Pay to the order of..." on the cheque. The name of the payee should be written out in full. The payee must endorse (or sign) the cheque in order to make the cheque negotiable.

The *endorsement* serves as a transfer of ownership of the funds that are being paid. The payee should endorse the cheque by using the same name as in the payee section of the cheque. In other words, if a cheque is payable to Susan Smith it should be endorsed in the same manner and not as Susy Smith.

Endorsement is usually made on the back, left end of the cheque. A cheque signed simply with the name on the face of the cheque has a blanket endorsement and is freely negotiable. A restrictive endorsement may be made with a rubber stamp that reads "Deposit only to the credit of Dr. D. Kay, Account # 1234-5678." This type of endorsement makes the cheque non-negotiable except for deposit to the named account.

EXHIBIT 14.1 **SAMPLE CHEQUE**

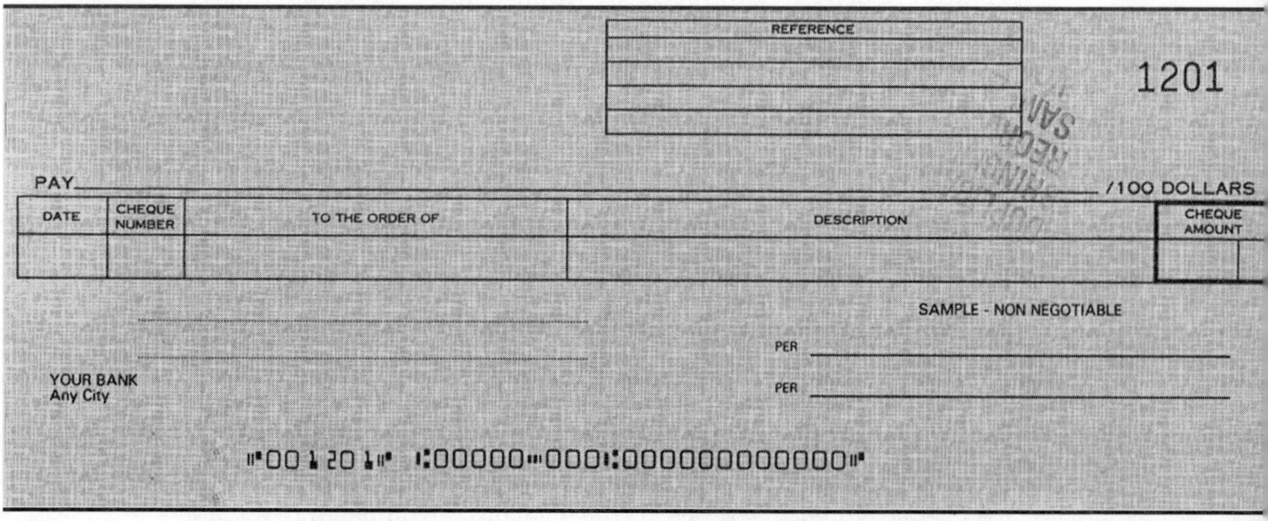

Reproduced with permission by Safeguard Business Systems, Inc., Fort Washington, PA 19034

EXHIBIT 14.2 **RESTRICTIVE ENDORSEMENT**

DEPOSIT ONLY TO THE CREDIT OF:
DR. I. TOOTH
123456-777

The *cheque writer* is the person from whose account the funds will be withdrawn. The cheque writer must sign the cheque on the signature line. Cheques must be written carefully and accurately in order to prevent error or fraud.

The *body* of the cheque contains the amount of the cheque written in words and the *figures* confirm that amount in numbers. The date on the cheque should be the same as the date it is issued. If a cheque is future dated or postdated, that means that the funds are not to be issued until that date. A cheque is considered stale dated and therefore invalid if it is older than six months. Bank or financial institution employees will ensure that every cheque that is negotiated contains the appropriate and accurate information in the body, date, figure, and signature areas on the cheque.

Cheque Ledger

The cheque ledger is the part of the chequebook where a record of all cheques issued and deposits made to the account are listed and a continuous balance is kept.

The cheque ledger entry (usually on the cheque stub) should be made before writing the cheque to ensure that funds are available to cover the cheque. The cheque ledger entry should include the date that the cheque was written, the cheque number, the name of the payee, the amount, and the purpose of the cheque.

All cheques received should be endorsed immediately with a restrictive endorsement stamp. Cheques, cash, and credit card slips should be kept locked in a drawer or cash box at all times. Regular daily bank deposits should be made so that large amounts of cash are not left in the office overnight where there is risk of robbery.

Corrections

If mistakes happen when writing a cheque, the word *void* should be written through the cheque ledger entry and a new cheque should be issued. The voided cheque should be kept with the chequebook. It is also advisable to tear off the signature portion of the cheque for added

EXHIBIT 14.3 CHEQUE LEDGER (STUB)

```
                           0001
                                                    19
                              BALANCE
                              FORWARD

        TO


        RE:
        GST AMOUNT          CHEQUE
                            AMOUNT
        GST #

        PST AMOUNT
                            DEPOSITS
        PST #
                            DEPOSITS

                            BALANCE
```

Reproduced with permission by Safeguard Business Systems, Inc., Fort Washington, PA 19034

security. Cheques should never be written in pencil or erasable ink. Never use correction fluid on a cheque; it will be considered non-negotiable.

NSF Cheques

A cheque that has been written for more than the amount that is in the account will be returned to the payee marked NSF (not sufficient funds). Accurate bookkeeping is essential to avoid the embarrassment of a returned cheque, also known as a returned item. If a cheque is returned due to insufficient funds, the payee will no longer trust the issuer of the cheque and this may affect the delivery of needed supplies.

The dental office administrator should always maintain a running balance of the account by recording all cheques that are written, all bank deposits, and any regular debits such as loan payments that are automatically withdrawn from the account. A diary card is useful to identify when these will be withdrawn. The administrator can then record the debits on the appropriate day, while maintaining a financial picture that is as accurate as possible.

Stop Payments

The issuer of a cheque can stop payment on it by written request to the bank. The stop payment order must include all relevant information such as the number of the cheque, date issued, name of payee, amount of the cheque, and the reason for stopping payment. It must also be signed by the issuer and reach the bank before the cheque is presented for payment. If the cheque has been previously negotiated, it is too late to stop the payment.

BANK DEPOSITS

A deposit slip is an itemized memorandum of the currency, cheques, and credit card payment summaries that are taken to the bank to be credited to the business account. All deposit slips must be legible and contain the correct date, the name and address of the depositor, and the account number. All cash is listed together under currency. Cheques are listed separately, usually by the last name and initial of the issuer of the cheque. When everything has been entered on the deposit slip, it is totalled and rechecked for accuracy.

The amount of the bank deposit slip must match the amount of payments received on the daily journal sheet. On the One Write daysheet, the amount of money received will appear in column B. (See p.131 in Chapter 11.)

Bank deposits should be made daily. If convenient, the administrator should go to the bank during a quiet period of the business day. Night depositories can be used, but deposits should not be made alone or according to a regular schedule. Robberies can occur if this routine is too predictable.

PAYMENT OPTIONS

Dental patients can choose from a variety of payment options, such as cash, cheque, or credit card. Some patients may wish to leave a post-dated cheque to allow time for the insurance payment to be received. All payments must be entered on the account ledger card and on the daily journal page. Payments received by mail are entered in the same manner as those made in person. Patients making cash or cheque payments must always be given a receipt.

Credit Card Payments

Many dental patients will choose to pay their account using a credit card, such as MasterCard or VISA. This form of payment is offered as

EXHIBIT 14.4 DEPOSIT SLIP

CHEQUES			CURRENT ACCOUNT DEPOSIT		
DETAILS	AMOUNT		CREDIT DR. I. TOOTH		
Doe, J	200	—			
Brown, S	100	—	DATE April 6.		
Smith, R	430	—	ACCOUNT NUMBER 123456-777		
			X 1		
			3 X 2	6	—
			2 X 5	10	—
			4 X 10	40	—
			5 X 20	100	—
			X 50		
			X 100		
			COIN		
			$	156	—
			CHEQUES	730	—
TOTALS FORWARD	730	—	NET DEPOSIT $	886	—

a convenience to patients to allow time for insurance payments to arrive. If the insurance form is submitted correctly, the insurance cheque should be received before interest charges are applied to the credit card account.

The dentist will make the necessary arrangements for this service through the bank. A transaction fee is charged for this service, varying from 1 percent to 5 percent of the total fee submitted. The bank will provide all of the necessary supplies including an imprinter, credit card slips, summary slips, and a merchant card. To verify that a credit card is valid, the administrator must call the credit card processing facility for authorization. When calling, you should be prepared with the merchant number, card number, expiry date, and the amount of the transaction.

The bank will provide a list of lost and stolen cards regularly. It is essential that the office administrator verify the signature as well as the expiry date on the card. To prepare credit card slips for deposit, each credit card transaction is itemized on a summary slip. The merchant's fee (service charge) is deducted from the total and the net amount is entered on the deposit slip.

BANK RECONCILIATION

The monthly bank statement will identify all of the financial transactions that occurred in the business account for the previous month and will be sent with all of the cancelled cheques. A cancelled cheque is one that has cleared the bank.

The statement is usually received at the beginning of the month, after the previous month's disbursements journal has been balanced and closed off. The bank statement will provide an area to reconcile the transactions or to verify that the business account figures agree with the bank.

Steps to Reconciliation

1. When the bank statement arrives, the administrator should arrange the cancelled cheques in numerical order and check off each cheque on the statement and the disbursements journal. Place a check mark next to all of the items that have cleared the bank.
2. Circle any items on the bank statement that do not appear on the disbursements journal, for example, bank interest, automatic debits, and NSF charges.
3. Record separately the cheques and deposits that do not appear on the bank statement. These items are outstanding because, although they do not appear on the statement, the funds have been designated.
4. Beginning with the bank balance that appears last on the statement, subtract the outstanding cheques.
5. Arrange the deposit slips in chronological order and tally the deposits made against those listed on the bank statement, ensuring that all amounts are recorded. List any deposits that have not cleared as outstanding deposits.
6. Add the outstanding deposits to the bank balance. This is the *adjusted bank balance.*

7. On the disbursements journal, or in the stub section of the cheque-book, subtract any bank charges that have been circled on the statement.

8. Subtract any automatic debit charges that have not been recorded on the disbursements journal.

The total becomes the *adjusted journal balance*.

The adjusted bank balance and the adjusted journal balance should match.

If the Reconciliation Does Not Balance

1. Calculate the amount of the difference. Review the bank statement, disbursements journal, cheque ledger stubs, and bank reconciliation.

2. Check the addition and subtraction of deposits and cheques.

3. Check the addition of the outstanding cheques.

TABLE 14.1 **SAMPLE BANK RECONCILIATION**

Bank balance (as per statement)				$5, 550.10
Subtract outstanding (O/S) cheques:				
#134	$ 75.00			
#251	277.01			
#139	135.00	Total O/S cheques	$487.01	5,063.09
Add outstanding (O/S) deposits				
June 4	$3,051.03			
ADJUSTED BANK BALANCE				$8,114.12
Journal balance				$8,268.66
Subtract bank charges:				
loan interest	$75.68			
NSF cheque	53.86			
service charge	25.00			
Total charges	$154.54			
ADJUSTED JOURNAL BALANCE				$8,114.12

EXHIBIT 14.5 SAMPLE BANK STATEMENT

HOME TOWN BANK
123 BANK STREET
CALGARY, ALBERTA
K8K 9K9

balance from previous statement $10,575.20

Date	Description	Dr.	Cr.	Balance
08/4/95	cheque # 1	108.00		10,467.20
10/4/95	cheque # 3	263.00		10,204.20
14/4/95	cheque # 4	271.25		9,932.95
20/4/95	loan int.	100.00		9,932.95
20/4/95	service charge	18.65		9,814.30

4. Check that the amounts are correctly entered on cheques and the cheque ledger and that they have been deducted correctly.
5. Check to ensure that the correct balance has been carried forward from one cheque stub to the next.
6. Recheck all calculations.
7. Determine if the amount of the difference is divisible by nine. If so, it could be a transposition of figures. For example, 36 could be recorded as 62, or 68 as 86, etc.
8. If all else fails, consult the accountant.

ASSIGNMENT

1. Prepare the bank deposit slip with the following information:
   Deposit to the account of Dr. D. Kay, 123 Molar Road, Your City, Province and Postal Code. Account # 1456–9876.
   Currency $262.00 (consisting of 10 × $20.00, 5 × $10.00, 2 × $5.00, 1 × $2.00)

Cheques	Smith	$56.80
	Jones	75.97
	Holiday	112.97
	Samson	50.00
	VISA summary	1,001.00

   What is the total amount of the deposit? _____

DR. D. KAY, 123 MOLAR ROAD, ACCOUNT 1456-9876					
CHEQUES	AMOUNT		CASH		
			coin		
			×2		
			×5		
			×10		
			×20		
			TOTAL CASH		
			+ CHEQUES		
TOTAL CHEQUES			NET DEPOSIT		

2. The bank statement has just arrived. Using the previously recorded disbursements journal (from the assignment in Chapter 12, p.150) and the steps outlined in this chapter, balance your bank statement. The statement reads as follows:

HOME TOWN BANK
123 BANK STREET
CALGARY, ALBERTA
K8K 9K9

Balance from previous statement $10,575.20

Date	Description	Dr.	Cr.	Balance
08/4/95	cheque # 1	108.00		10,467.20
10/4/95	cheque # 2	263.00		10,204.20
14/4/95	cheque # 3	271.25		9,932.95
20/4/95	loan int.	100.00		9,932.95
20/4/95	service charge	18.65		9,814.30

CHAPTER FIFTEEN

RECORDS MANAGEMENT

OBJECTIVE

At the end of this chapter, the student will be able to identify and describe the following: alphabetic and numeric filing systems, the steps to proper filing and storage of files, hazards of filing systems, a regular purging system, laws concerning dental records, and how to find a "lost" chart.

TOPICS

- confidentiality
- informed consent
- separating clinical and financial information
- purging charts, storing inactive charts
- fire and theft protection
- making appropriate chart entries and corrections
- identifying medical alerts
- types of filing systems
- steps in filing alphabetically and numerically
- colour coding charts for fast retrieval
- storage cabinets and equipment
- potential workplace safety hazards

IMPORTANCE OF CONFIDENTIALITY

Maintaining accurate records in the dental office is an important responsibility of the dental team in general. In a dental office there are two basic types of recorded information:

1. Clinical records
2. Financial records

The clinical record, referred to as the chart, consists of complete and accurate information regarding the patient's dental health as well as a thorough medical history.

The financial records include the financial information on each patient as well as the business records for the office. These records are referred to as the accounts receivable and accounts payable. All records must be protected against loss and/or damage.

The accurate administration of dental office records will help to ensure that every patient is provided with the best possible care, and that the dentist is protected against unnecessary legal action. Protecting the confidential nature of all records within the office is the responsibility of the dental office administrator. A dedicated dental professional will recognize the legal implications of his or her work as well as the importance of confidentiality. A patient's record must never be discussed with an unauthorized person. No question should be asked about a patient in front of another patient. All communications with the dentist or other dental team members should be conducted in private, out of the hearing of other patients.

Every patient is legally and ethically entitled to privacy. It is the responsibility of the dental team to uphold and protect that right. Dental professionals are in the unique position of knowing a great deal of information about a patient, including his or her medical history. The patient must feel assured that all information given will remain confidential. Otherwise, the patient may withhold critical information which could affect the quality of the care provided and could also expose other patients and the health care providers to health risks.

RECORDS PROTECTION

Many dental offices are designed with a raised front counter or window to provide protection of confidential records. A private consultation area that is away from patients waiting in the reception area is helpful. The pegboard accounting system has been designed to protect confidentiality by closing easily when not in use.

Records can be stored in lockable filing cabinets made of fireproof material. The destruction or loss of records through fire or other catastrophe can seriously handicap a practice. To protect clinical and financial records,

- Be careful not to leave records where they can be seen.
- Never leave records out of their appropriate file space. When finished using a record, return it to its proper place.
- When leaving for the day, be certain all records are protected in file cabinets and/or storage units.
- If records are temporarily removed from the office, perhaps by the dentist, they should be replaced with a folder that is signed and dated. This provides an audit trail to track misplaced charts.
- Collect the charts periodically from the treatment rooms. The dental assistant, hygienist, or dentist will usually bring the chart to the front counter; however, it is a good idea to check from time to time to ensure that you have proper control over all of the records.
- If you have a computer, ensure that a backup procedure is done daily. Backup tapes should be stored in a fireproof safe. Lock the computer so that no one can access information at night.
- When patient information is displayed on the computer screen, ensure that the screen is adjusted so that other patients cannot see the information.

RETENTION OF RECORDS

Some authorities recommend that patient records be retained forever. However, legally a dental office need only to retain records for six to seven years. Many dentists will opt to retain inactive charts in a separate storage area, perhaps at an outside facility. A patient's file is usually considered to be inactive when the patient has not returned to the office in a period of two years and several attempts have been made to recall the patient to the practice. No record should ever be destroyed or discarded without specific permission from the dentist and in accordance with the office policy. A continuing system of purging old charts will help to reduce the time spent attempting to follow up on inactive files.

Inactive records can also be stored on microfilm to reduce storage space. A large number of dental records can be photographed on small strips of film, then the record stored in an archive file and retrieved if necessary. A microfilmed document may be viewed through a large viewer called a microfiche projector.

RELEASE OF INFORMATION

Any information regarding a patient should not be released from the office without first obtaining a written release of information. Insurance companies will frequently call the dental office requesting information regarding a dental claim. It is permissible to release only the specific information that pertains to the claim in question. It is advisable to take the number of the dental claims adjudicator and call back to verify that it is, in fact, an insurance company inquiry. When a patient signs the dental insurance form, the caption above the signature may read as follows:

> I understand that the fees listed in this claim may not be covered by or may exceed my plan benefits. I understand that I am financially responsible to my dentist for the entire treatment. I acknowledge that the total fee of $____ is accurate and has been charged to me for services rendered. I authorize release of the information contained in this claim form to my insuring company/plan administrator.

In addition to verifying that the patient understands the fees and accepts responsibility for payment, this clause provides written authorization to release information to an insurance company regarding that claim.

INFORMED CONSENT

In order to give informed consent, the patient must be informed of the proposed treatment, cost, and risk factors associated with each dental procedure. It is unrealistic to obtain a signed consent form for each and every dental procedure; however, it is a wise measure to protect the doctor against malpractice litigation.

Children under 18 years of age must have a consent form signed by the parent or guardian to authorize the dental office to perform necessary dental procedures and, in particular, administer anaesthesia. A general consent form that encompasses all aspects of dental treatment may be included with the new patient registration form.

THE CLINICAL RECORD

Clinical records are legal documents and may subpoenaed to be used in a court of law or even for forensic identification. All information must

EXHIBIT 15.1 **SAMPLE CONSENT CLAUSE**

I hereby consent to the performing of the dental and oral surgery procedures necessary or advisable for my dental health, including the administration of local or general anaesthesia, as outlined to me. I accept
responsibility for the fees charged and have read this statement and understand the contents.

Signed _____Witness _____

Date _____

be complete, accurate, and legible. Comments made to the patient by
the dentist should also be recorded to protect the dentist legally. Any
instructions that were given to the patient but failed to be carried out
should be recorded. Test results to confirm clinical findings and also
kept in the chart along with an outline or plan for future treatment.

A clinical record may typically contain:

1. A patient registration form. This may include limited financial
   information necessary to complete the patient information portion
   of an insurance claim form.
2. A thorough medical and dental history, including information concerning the patient's health, past history, allergies, and current
   medications.
3. Examination and treatment records, which include all treatment
   provided in the practice and a record of any prescriptions written
   for the patient.
4. Radiographs may be stored with the chart or maintained in a separate file.
5. All correspondence regarding that patient.

See Exhibits 15.2 and 15.3 for examples of clinical records. All
entries that are recorded on the patient's chart should be legible. An
error on a chart entry should never be erased. Make corrections by
crossing through the previous entry and initialling the correction.

Patient records are kept together in a file folder or envelope and
may be filed alphabetically or numerically. Most dental offices file their
patient records alphabetically. However, a computerized identification
number may be assigned to each chart for the purpose of cross refer-
encing. Files may be colour coded to make filing and retrieval easier
and faster. Tabs that combine colours and letters are used to identify

EXHIBIT 15.2 **REGISTRATION FORM**

WELCOME TO OUR DENTAL OFFICE

(For office use only)

I.D. #

MEDICAL ALERT

Date _____

Your co-operation in completing this questionnaire is essential to providing you with the highest standard of dental care. All information is strictly confidential and will remain with this office. Our receptionist is available to assist you with the completion of this form. **PLEASE PRINT.**

REGISTRATION INFORMATION

The patient is an: Adult ☐ Child ☐ Adult under guardianship ☐ Name of Guardian: _____

Name: (last) _____ (first) _____ (initial) _____

Dr. ☐ Mr. ☐ Mrs. ☐ Ms. ☐ Miss ☐

Address: (street) _____ (apt.#) _____ (city) _____ (province) _____ (postal code) _____

Reason for today's visit? Examination ☐ Emergency ☐ Other ☐ _____

Is there a dental problem you would like treated immediately? _____ Preferred appt. time? _____

Home Phone: (   ) _____ Driver's Lic. No. _____ S.I.N. _____

Bus. Phone: (   ) _____ Ext. ____ Employer: _____ May we call you at work? ☐

PERSONAL INFORMATION

Prefers to be called: _____ Occupation: _____

Date of Birth: M___D___Y___ Age: ____ Sex: ____ Marital Status: ____ Name of Spouse: _____

Are other family members patients at our office? Yes ☐ Names: _____

Whom may we thank for referring you? _____

MEDICAL PRIORITY

Family Physician: _____ Phone: (   ) _____

Medical Specialist: _____ Phone: (   ) _____
(if presently under care)

In case of emergency, please contact: _____ Phone: (   ) _____

Nearest relative not living with you: _____ Phone: (   ) _____

FINANCIAL INFORMATION

Person responsible for account: Self ☐   Spouse ☐   Other ☐   **Please complete all information if different than above.**

Name: (last) _____ (first) _____ (initial) _____ Phone: (   ) _____

Address: (street) _____ (apt.#) _____ (city) _____ (province) _____ (postal code) _____

Employed by: _____ Phone: (   ) _____

Driver's Lic. No. _____ S.I.N. _____

PRIMARY DENTAL INSURANCE		SECONDARY DENTAL INSURANCE	
Subscriber's name:	D.O.B.	Subscriber's name:	D.O.B.
Emp./Grp. policy holder:	Ins. yr. end	Emp./Grp. policy holder:	Ins. yr. end
Ins. Co.	Tel.	Ins. Co.	Tel.
Grp./Ind. policy No.	Cert. No.	Grp./Ind. policy No.	Cert. No.
I.D./S.I.N.	Max. Coverage.	I.D./S.I.N.	Max. Coverage.
% coverage: Basic Maj. Rest. Ortho. Other Other		% coverage: Basic Maj. Rest. Ortho. Other Other	

METHOD OF PAYMENT (For office use only)   **CASH** ☐   **CHEQUE** ☐   **CREDIT CARD** ☐   **OTHER** ☐

PATIENT REGISTRATION   DENTAL HISTORY

The DMD (Dental Management Document) and the DMD Emergency Treatment System have been reproduced with the permission of Dental Risk Management Systems Inc., which holds the copyright.

EXHIBIT 15.3 **PATIENT PROGRESS FORM**

MEDICAL ALERT	CONDITION	PREMEDICATION	ALLERGIES	ANAEST.

PROGRESS NOTES

Patient: _____ Dentist: _____

55	54	53	52	51	18	17	16	15	14	13	12	11	21	22	23	24	25	26	27	28	61	62	63	64	65

R   L

85	84	83	82	81	48	47	46	45	44	43	42	41	31	32	33	34	35	36	37	38	71	72	73	74	75

DATE	Tooth No.	Procedure Code	Surface	Anaesthetic Used	TREATMENT COMMENTS	X-Ray Log	Initial	FEE

PROGRESS NOTES   **PROGRESS NOTES**

The DMD (Dental Management Document) and the DMD Emergency Treatment System have been reproduced with the permission of Dental Risk Management Systems Inc., which holds the copyright.

the first two letters of the patient's last name. A coding system makes it easier to spot a misfiled chart and aids fast and efficient filing and chart retrieval.

Medical Histories

A complete and thorough medical history should be obtained before treating every patient. In order to provide the best possible care, a dentist must be aware of any risk factors that may impede treatment or cause an unexpected patient response. The dentist must also be prepared to protect him or herself and the dental team from exposure to an infectious disease that can be transferred to other patients. The sterilization procedures may also need to be considered.

Many dental office administrators will allow the patient to complete his or her own medical history. Some patients may not feel that certain questions are relevant and may skim over them. It is advisable to review important questions with the patient to avoid risk during treatment. Any condition considered to be a medical alert should be underlined or otherwise indicated in red on the patient's chart. The dentist may wish to conduct further investigation about the medical condition before proceeding with treatment. A patient seen on an emergency basis poses the highest risk if time is not provided to elicit the necessary medical history.

FINANCIAL RECORDS

Financial records such as insurance forms and financial information regarding the patient's account do not belong in the chart with the clinical information. Instead, these items are secured separately. Ledger cards are generally used for this purpose and stored alphabetically in a vertical ledger tray. These trays have a spring mechanism to hold the cards tightly when not in use. Account ledger cards record all the charges, fees, and payments made for each family.

Business records are usually stored using a subject file system. Each file is separated into specific categories such as "laboratory expenses" and "business office supplies." Business records include unpaid bills, expense records, payroll records, business correspondence, cancelled cheques, bank statements, record of income and expenses, and financial statements with tax records.

An efficient system of records management will provide the dental professional with

- fast retrieval of information
- legal protection
- protection of confidentiality
- reduction of unnecessary records and wasted space
- the ability to provide the best possible dental care

FILING SYSTEMS

Equipment

Filing is the organization, protection, and control of records. Before purchasing filing equipment and supplies, consideration should be given to the type of records to be filed, the space available, and the budget for filing purposes. The equipment that is selected should be practical as well as providing protection and proper storage of records. Fire protection is important and all storage cabinets should lock. Confidentiality, retrieval speed, and the cost of space and equipment are just a few issues to be considered.

Many offices use a vertical drawer file system, which contains hanging files. Each chart cover has a plastic guide that allows it to hang on the guides in the drawers. Open-shelf filing is becoming increasingly popular. Colour coding in an open-shelf filing system along with index guides help to quickly identify a misplaced chart.

Equipment Safety

Serious accidents can occur in any work setting, and the front desk area of a dental office is no exception. Filing equipment can be a major cause of injuries if it is not used properly. Dental records (charts) become rather heavy when they contain clinical records, radiographs, correspondence, etc. If too much weight is distributed to the top shelves of any filing system, it will become top heavy and could fall over. This can be avoided if the bottom drawers are heavier than the top. In addition, when a file is pulled out from a drawer, the drawer should be closed immediately. This will help to maintain the balance of the filing system.

Drawers should be kept closed when not in use to prevent injury to someone who may wish to obtain a file from a lower drawer and may hurt themselves by bumping into a top drawer that was left ajar. Bottom drawers left open can cause employees to trip, leading to serious injury to themselves and others.

Filing

Filing is the act of classifying and arranging records so that they will be preserved safely and can be retrieved quickly when needed. An alphabetical filing system is by far the easiest and most commonly used system for filing patient records. In alphabetical filing, all items are filed in alphabetical order following the basic rules of indexing.

A numerical system identifies each chart or document by an assigned number. Numerical filing systems are commonly used in large group practices. A numerical filing system provides a more even distribution of charts in the files. Items can be located using a cross-referencing system in which each item is listed in alphabetical order, by name and document number.

A chronological file is divided into months and may be further subdivided into days of the month. This kind of file may be used for the dental recall system or as a reminder system for miscellaneous tasks, such as routine maintenance.

The basic rules of filing are as follows:

1. Keep the filing system simple. The simpler the system, the easier it is to work with. For most practices, alphabetical filing with colour coding is the simplest and most efficient method.
2. Leave adequate working space in each file. Papers tightly wedged into the file slow the filing process and make records hard to find. This also increases the risk of damage to filed materials. Leave at least four inches of working space on each shelf or drawer.
3. Label shelves or drawers (if possible). It is easier to go directly to the proper file area if all files are clearly, neatly, and accurately labelled as to the contents.
4. Clearly label folders. Each file folder should have a neatly typed label showing the patient's full name. This saves you from going through the chart to make certain that you have the correct patient file.
5. Use out-guides. An out-guide is like a bookmark for the filing system. When a folder is removed from the file, place an out-guide to mark its place. This makes it faster to return records to the file and easy to spot where records are missing.

6. Presort folders into approximate order before starting to file to speed the filing process.

Colour coded purge tabs or labels make it easier to sort records into active and inactive categories.

Steps to Filing

1. *Condition the file.* If the file is tattered and worn, prepare a new chart cover/file folder and transfer the information from the old chart cover. Remember to place tabs and labels in the correct locations.

2. *Index.* Choose the caption under which a record is to be filed. Last names should be typed on the chart first. Hyphenated surnames are considered to be one name. For example, Mary Brown-Smith would be filed under B. Each surname is considered to be a single important element when alphabetizing.

   For example,

   > S M I T H , J O E
   > SMITH, MARY
   > SMITHERS, ANNA

   If the first word in a compound surname is abbreviated, it is indexed as if written out.

   For example,

   > STJOHN, GILDA
   > ST.JOHN, KAREN
   > ST. JOHN, MAX
   > SAINT JOHN, RICHARD

   If you look in a telephone book under St. John, a cross reference notation will direct you to *Saint.* Titles, degrees, and seniority designations are disregarded when indexing, as in Capt. James Blueberry, Rev. W.R. Rogers, Joe Smith Sr., and Joe Smith Jr. Take some time to examine how indexing is done in the telephone book and follow the standard rules consistently.

3. *Code the chart* with the appropriate colours or tabs for fast retrieval. Colour coding saves time and improves accuracy.

4. *Cross reference.* If you are using a complex system or a combination of filing systems, be sure to cross reference. It is also a good idea to insert a blank chart under an unusually spelled last name. For example, if the name sounds like "Vice" but is actually spelled "Weiscz," place an empty folder in the V-file with a cross reference to the W-file:

   > VICE, Mr. Tom (see WEISZ).

5. *Sort*. Presorting is arranging the files in the order of the filing sequence. This process saves time and also helps to prevent a back injury from continuous bending up and down.
6. *File and store* the records.

There is no such thing as a lost chart!

An efficient filing system that is simple to use and easily understood by all staff members will prevent wasted time trying to find a misplaced chart. Remember that all office records are legal documents and must be protected and filed properly. If any staff member who is not familiar with the filing system attempts to be helpful by filing for you, make sure that he or she is familiar with the system and will follow all of the necessary steps.

A systematic plan for the proper storage and retrieval of records will save time. All records must be available for easy reference. The needs of the office and the space available for equipment will determine what the most appropriate system will be for that office. Developing a positive attitude about such a responsible task will be helpful for the dental office administrator.

ASSIGNMENT

1. Describe the information that is usually included in the patient's chart.
2. Where should financial records be kept?
3. What information is recorded on ledger cards?
4. What is meant by "release of information"?
5. What are the two basic types of records in the office?
6. Describe an example of a cross reference system.
7. What are active files? Describe briefly.

CHAPTER SIXTEEN

PREVENTIVE DENTISTRY AND PATHOLOGY

OBJECTIVE

At the end of this chapter, the student will be able to identify and describe the following: the role of sugar in cariogenesis, the formation of plaque and colonization of bacteria, nutritional requirements for maintaining oral health, common dental pathologies, and preventive programs.

TOPICS

- role of the dental office administrator in a preventive program
- relationship between nutrition and oral health
- personal oral health
- formation of plaque
- relationship between carbohydrates and plaque
- flossing
- toothbrushing techniques
- mechanics of a dental recall appointment
- pathology

PREVENTIVE DENTISTRY

Successful businesses depend on repeat business to maintain viability, and dentistry is no different. A program of dental prevention and maintenance helps to circumvent the need for more extensive and costly procedures through the early diagnosis and treatment of dental disease. Preventive dentistry can reduce the financial burden to the patient that is associated with dental treatment by treating minor problems before they require more comprehensive procedures. Many patients will wait until something hurts before they will seek treatment. This costs them time and money. Dental disease can damage physical well-being, create psychological trauma, and cause a loss of wages to the dental patient.

Decayed teeth can lead to infections throughout the body, and decayed or missing teeth can interfere with proper nutrition, leading to disorders of digestion. Conversely, poor nutrition can cause dental disease, creating a continuous cycle of ill health.

The mouth is one of the most important instruments for communication. Speech impairments can be treated and often prevented. The smile is one of the most powerful ways to communicate, especially when it is aesthetically pleasing and free of disease and odour. Unsightly teeth or bad breath can affect the self-esteem and personality of the patient.

Healthy Teeth for a Lifetime

Preventive dentistry helps to maintain oral structures for the longest time possible. When properly cared for, the teeth and surrounding structures should last for a lifetime. All members of the dental team should share this philosophy of preventive care and demonstrate it every day. A program of personal oral hygiene and good nutritional habits is necessary for good physical and oral health. Every dental team member should ensure that all personal dental work is completed and that his or her oral health is optimal, reflecting the health conscious image of the office.

Patient Education

Patient education can help achieve optimal dental health and reduce the financial and psychological burden of dental treatment. A patient education program will include nutritional counselling and a personal oral hygiene program for plaque control. Patients must be encouraged to be willing and active participants in their own dental health and to understand that dental decay is entirely preventable.

Patients must be motivated to return for regular preventive treatment, which will include professional prophylaxis (cleaning), an examination, and oral hygiene instructions or reinforcement. Dental x-rays may be taken to detect underlying problems that are not visible to the naked eye. Fluoride treatments are often routinely given to children. The dental office administrator should be familiar with the procedures that are followed during every preventive appointment in order to communicate effectively with patients. Patients must be educated about the importance of scheduling routine visits and keeping their appointments.

Pit and Fissure Sealants

A preventive procedure for children between the ages of 6 and 12 years is the placement of pit and fissure sealants on the first and second molars as they erupt into the dentition. The sealants application is a noninvasive procedure that protects susceptible areas before decay has an opportunity to begin. The occlusal pits and the fissures, or grooves, are difficult areas to cleanse with normal brushing, leaving them prone to decay. This procedure may be done on adult bicuspids and the lingual surfaces of anterior teeth if the pits and fissures are deep. If these areas are left unprotected, decay could form and a more invasive procedure, such as an amalgam or composite filling, may be required.

The dental office administrator plays a crucial role in creating and maintaining a preventive program by continuously reinforcing the importance of treatment and follow-up, and motivating the patient to return for future care. It is important also to evaluate home care procedures.

A patient education program is effective only if the patient truly believes that the dental staff care about his or her dental, physical, and emotional well-being. Thus, the patient shares the office philosophy of preventive care and becomes an active participant.

CAUSES OF DENTAL DISEASE

The causes of tooth decay are not completely understood, but certain facts are known. Tooth decay is associated with refined foods and the ingestion of various forms of sugars and starch. There is no cure for tooth decay. Prevention is the only real answer to the problem. This includes cleanliness and the removal of plaque.

The Formation of Plaque

One of the forerunners of dental caries (decay) is plaque. Plaque is a gummy mass of micro-organisms that grows on the crowns and spreads along the roots of teeth. It is a colourless, soft, thin film consisting of food debris, dead epithelial cells, bacteria, saliva, and mucus. This film provides a medium for the growth of various forms of bacteria. Plaque plays an important role in the development of dental decay and periodontal and gingival diseases. Calcified plaque forms dental calculus, commonly referred to as tartar.

Plaque is almost always present in the mouth and begins to form less than one minute after brushing. Ingested nutrients and soluble sugars easily diffuse into the plaque. If the bacteria remain on the teeth they will begin to form colonies. The action of the bacteria on sugars and starches creates lactic acid, which can quickly and permanently dissolve tooth enamel. The acid is produced just half an hour after sugar comes into contact with the plaque. It is for this reason that sweet or starchy foods are so harmful between meals and at bedtime. The teeth should be thoroughly brushed and rinsed after eating.

Once plaque has been properly removed, it takes 24 hours for the bacteria to colonize. Brushing the teeth will disturb the colonies of bacteria, thus neutralizing the harmful cariogenous process. The teeth should be thoroughly brushed at least once a day and preferably after every meal. Dental floss or tape should be used to remove any particles of food from the interproximal spaces. If teeth can not be brushed after every meal, the mouth should be thoroughly rinsed with water.

NUTRITION AND ORAL HEALTH

Diet plays an important part in the prevention of tooth decay. Sugars and starches should be limited, especially between meals. This applies particularly to those which are sticky and tend to cling to the teeth. For example, raisins are sticky and contain concentrated natural sugar. Chewable vitamin tablets, particularly vitamin C, contain ascorbic acid, which will destroy the enamel of the tooth. The mouth should be thoroughly rinsed with water following ingestion of a chewable vitamin.

Decay that is not treated will progress through the tooth enamel and the dentin just below it into the pulp of the tooth, which contains the nerves. When it reaches the pulp, it can cause intense pain. Enamel that has been destroyed does not regenerate. The decay must be removed and the cavity filled. When decay has reached the pulp of a tooth, it may be necessary to perform root canal therapy or extract the tooth.

Fluoride

The development of dental decay can be decreased significantly by drinking water that contains fluoride or by the topical application of fluoride. The level of fluoride in controlled water fluoridation is so low that there is no danger of ingesting an acutely toxic quantity of fluoride from water. The fluoride concentration for drinking water is approximately one part per million parts of water (1 mg/1000 mL).

Even in communities where fluoride is added to the water supply, a dentist may choose to apply a fluoride solution directly to a child's teeth. Many dentists will include this process with each child's recall visit. Fluoride drops or tablets may also be prescribed in small amounts, but this treatment must always be carefully supervised by a dentist or doctor.

Fluoride is effective in lowering the incidence of dental caries. It is absorbed in small quantities and stored in the bones of developing teeth. The teeth serve as storage sites for fluoride, with the highest concentration found in the outer surface of the enamel.

Toothbrushing Techniques

A toothbrush should be flexible and easily manipulated. It should be cleaned and left to dry after each usage. Most dentists recommend soft bristles to prevent damage to the soft tissues of the oral cavity, which can result from improper or vigorous brushing. Hard bristles can cause abrasion, recession of the gingival margin, and sensitivity.

A toothbrush should be impervious to moisture, durable, and easily replaced. Toothbrushes not only disturb the colonies of bacteria on teeth, but they can also harbour bacteria and become a breeding ground for germs. Toothbrushes should be replaced at least once every three months. Dentifrice or toothpaste aids in cleaning and polishing tooth surfaces. Those containing fluorides or baking soda provide added protection to the teeth.

A plaque control program should meet the needs of the individual patient. The toothbrushing technique should be evaluated and instructions clearly communicated to the patient on every recall visit.

There are various techniques for toothbrushing. The dental hygienist or the dentist will select the method that is most suitable for a patient based on his or her manual dexterity and current oral hygiene.

Although there are some minor differences, all of the techniques include introducing the angled bristles into the gingival sulcus of the tooth to disturb the bacterial colonies. The sulcus is the space between the free gingiva and the tooth. The depth of a healthy sulcus rarely exceeds 2.5 mm. The gingival papilla is the interdental extension of the free gingiva. The gingival sulcus traps bacterial plaque that, when calcified, becomes calculus. Calculus must be removed by the dental hygienist with a scaling instrument.

Along with sulcus brushing, some of the methods will incorporate a gum massage. This helps the blood circulate through the soft tissue. Some toothbrushes have a rubber stimulator tip attached for gum massage and stimulation of tissue. Normal healthy gingiva should surround the tooth to support it, should be firm and resistant, tightly attached to the bone or tooth, and salmon pink in colour.

All toothbrushing techniques will provide cleansing action for three tooth surfaces. The interproximal surfaces must be cleaned separately with dental floss. Flossing done on a regular basis will disorganize the colonies of bacteria and help in the prevention of tooth decay and gum disease.

THE RECALL APPOINTMENT

It is recommended that the dental office administrator observe the procedures involved in preventive recall appointments and as many other clinical procedures as possible. This will be helpful when discussing the appointment with the patient and understanding the clinical aspects of treatment. The administrator can assist the patient in knowing what to expect.

The preventive recall appointment consists of an oral examination, visual examination of the oral mucosa, and general hygiene. Periodontal pockets will be identified and charted along with any suspected carious lesions.

The dental hygienist or dentist will perform subgingival scaling if necessary to remove calculus or tartar. Radiographs may be necessary to detect interproximal decay that is not easily seen. The teeth are then polished (prophylaxis).

There are several methods of performing prophylaxis. A prophy-jet may be used, which cleans the coronal surfaces of the teeth with a high-powered warm water spray that contains a sodium compound to remove stains. The dental provider may prefer to use a rubber cup and prophy paste. The rubber cup attaches to a high speed handpiece and is dipped in a prophy or polishing paste containing finely ground pumice.

Some dental offices routinely perform fluoride treatments for patients up to the age of 18. Fluoride is available in many different flavours to make the process more pleasant for children. Fluoride is toxic if swallowed and care should be taken to ensure that the child does not swallow it during treatment. Small children may have a topical fluoride application either painted on the teeth or applied from a tray for three or four minutes. It is also available in the form of a rinse that is held in the mouth for one minute. The latter is not recommended for small children.

DENTAL PATHOLOGY

Gingivitis

Inflammation of the gingiva or gingivitis can occur as the result of dental neglect. It can also be an early sign of a vitamin deficiency, diabetes, or possible blood disorder. Occasionally, oral contraceptives can be linked to gingivitis. Gingivitis is characterized by inflammation of the gums with painless swelling. Symptoms may include redness of the mucosa, change of normal contours, bleeding, and periodontal pockets. The gums can become detached from the teeth as the infection spreads. The infection could spread to the alveolar process, causing resorption of the bone and resulting in very little support for the tooth structure. Treatment consists of removal of irritating factors such as calculus and plaque. Periodontal surgery may be required in severe cases.

Periodontitis

Periodontitis is a form of progressive gingivitis. It is also characterized by inflammation of the oral mucosa. Causes include poor oral hygiene and/or improper occlusion. It is the major cause of tooth loss after middle age.

Signs of periodontitis include acute onset of bright red gum inflammation, swelling of interdental papilla, or loosening of teeth, typically without inflammatory symptoms, progressing to the loss of teeth and the alveolar bone. Acute systemic infection, fever, or chills may accompany the symptoms.

Treatment includes scaling, root planing, curettage for infection control, and periodontal surgery to prevent recurrence. Good oral hygiene and frequent dental checkups are necessary in the management of this disease.

Necrotizing Ulcerative Gingivitis

Necrotizing ulcerative gingivitis is commonly known as trench mouth and is usually acute in nature. It is characterized by a bacterial infection of the mouth and can be caused by stress factors and systemic disease resistant factors such as poor oral hygiene, insufficient rest, nutritional deficiency, and smoking. Symptoms include sudden onset of painful superficial bleeding and gingival ulcers covered with a grey-white membrane. Malaise, mild fever, excessive salivation, bad breath, pain on swallowing or talking, and enlarged submaxillary lymph nodes are also symptomatic of this disease.

Treatment consists of removal of devitalized tissue with an ultrasonic cavitron. Antibiotics such as penicillin or erythromycin are administered by mouth for the infection. Analgesics are administered as needed. Treatment also includes hourly mouth rinses with equal amounts of hydrogen peroxide and warm water, a soft, nonirritating diet, rest, and cessation of smoking. Improvement is usually evident within 24 hours.

Glossitis

Glossitis is inflammation of the tongue. It may be caused by a streptococcal infection, irritation or injury, jagged teeth, ill fitting dentures, biting during convulsions, alcohol, spicy foods, smoking, sensitivity to toothpaste or mouthwash, Vitamin B deficiency, or anaemia. Glossitis is characterized by a reddened, ulcerated, or swollen tongue. This may cause an obstruction of the airway and painful chewing and swallowing. Speech becomes difficult with a painful tongue.

Treatment of the underlying cause is the preferred approach and may include topical anaesthetic mouthwash or systemic analgesics, such as aspirin and/or acetaminophen, for painful lesions. Good oral hygiene, regular dental checkups, vigorous chewing, along with the avoidance of hot, cold, or spicy foods and alcohol, are recommended therapies.

ASSIGNMENT

1. What is the primary goal of preventive dentistry?
2. How can preventive dentistry help to reduce the forms of dental neglect?
3. What is important for the dental health team involved in the preventive dentistry program?
4. Briefly describe plaque.
5. What does sugar do in relation to decay?
6. What are pit and fissure sealants?
7. What are the objectives in patient education for preventive dentistry?

CHAPTER SEVENTEEN

PHARMACOLOGY

OBJECTIVE

At the end of this chapter, the student will be able to identify and describe the following: how to read and translate a prescription, the reasons for premedication, some of the common prescriptions used in general practice including dosages, and special instructions to patients, potential side effects and drug interactions, and the components of a prescription.

TOPICS

- understanding the prescription
- abbreviations
- medications commonly prescribed
- narcotics control
- needs of special patients
- premedication
- dealing with the pharmacist

PRESCRIPTION DRUGS

Pharmacology is the study of the nature, preparation, administration, and effects of drugs. Drugs are introduced to the body to assist or enhance its natural physiological defence functions and to overcome disease or infection. Medications that are commonly prescribed in dentistry are

- analgesics
- anaesthetics
- sedatives
- antibiotics

The dental office administrator should become familiar with the types of drugs customarily prescribed and related procedures and should be alert to any possible side effects or interactions that may occur.

A **prescription** is a written order from a licensed medical doctor or dentist to a pharmacist. It contains specific information directing the pharmacist to dispense medication to a patient. The dentist is legally obliged to exercise "due care" when treating patients with medication. In addition to obtaining a complete medical history from the patient, including any allergic reactions or chronic health problems, a dentist must understand drugs and their properties, and must determine the most appropriate method of administration or introduction to the body.

Drug names can be divided into three main classes:

1. *Chemical name.* This is the base compound that is the main ingredient of the medication.
2. *Generic name.* This is usually a shortened form of the chemical name. Any manufacturer can use the generic name when marketing a drug. It is not capitalized.
3. *Brand name.* Brand named drugs are controlled by business firms and have registered trademarks. Brand names are always capitalized.

A drug manufacturer can distribute a generic name drug to several companies, who can then sell it under their own brand names. For example, ampicillin is the base compound for more than 200 brands of antibiotics. Generic medications are usually much less expensive than corresponding brand name drugs. In most cases, patients have the right to request generic substitutes. Many pharmacists will ask patients if they would prefer the generic substitute, unless otherwise directed to dispense only the brand name medication.

The Prescription

The prescription describes the medication to be taken and instructions for administration to the body.

The prescription consists of the following components:

1. The *heading* includes the name, address, and telephone number of the dentist; the name, address, and age of the patient; and the date of the prescription.

EXHIBIT 17.1 **SAMPLE PRESCRIPTION**

(1) Dr. D. Kay
123 Cuspid Court,
Winnipeg, Manitoba, M8J 9K9

Reg. # 394857676398404-87

Name of Patient:_____ Age _____

Address:_____

Rx (2)

(3) Fiorinal, 325 mg

(4) 24 capsules

(5) Sig: caps i q4h p.r.n. for pain

(6) Refill 2×   (7) _____

2. The *superscription* includes the symbol Rx. This represents a Latin abbreviation for the word recipe. It means "take thou" and is an order for the pharmacist to take the drugs listed and dispense them to the patient.

3. The *inscription* is the body of the prescription, which includes the name of the drug and the strength. In this example, the drug is Fiorinal (an analgesic) and the strength is 325 mg.

4. The *subscription* contains the volume and the amount of the drug to be dispensed. It will often include the word "dispense," followed by a number or a total volume. The doctor is recommending that the drug be dispensed in the form of tablets and the pharmacist should count 24.

5. *Signature* comes from the Latin word *signa* meaning "mark a label." This section may actually be preceded by the word "label." It includes specific instructions for the patient on how the preparation is to be used.

6. *Refill information* must be noted by the prescribing dentist to indicate the number of refills permitted.

7. The *signature* of the prescriber is the legal signature of the dentist, necessary on all prescriptions.

Prescriptions do not contain mysterious or secret messages. The symbols and phrases used on prescriptions are abbreviated Latin words. For example, p.r.n. means *pro re nata,* which is Latin for "as needed." Table 17.1 lists the English equivalents of Latin abbreviations that are frequently used in writing prescriptions.

Types of Drugs Commonly Prescribed

Analgesics are drugs used to relieve pain. The prefix *an* means without and the root word *algesia* means pain. They may be narcotic or non-narcotic. Mild analgesics, such as salicylate (Aspirin), acetaminophen (Tylenol), or ibuprofen (Motrin), for example, are used for headache and toothache. More potent analgesics that may induce stupor are narcotics, such morphine, codeine, or Percodan. Many analgesics contain codeine or other narcotics combined with analgesics which are non-narcotic, such as Tylenol 3 with codeine. Medications that contain a narcotic agent can be habit forming; therefore, they must be used with caution.

Anaesthetics are agents that reduce or eliminate sensation. The prefix *an* means without and the root word *aesthesia* means feeling or sensation. A local anaesthetic affects a particular region of the body. This is the most frequently used type of pain control in dentistry. Examples of local anaesthetic solutions are Xylocaine and Novocaine.

A general anaesthetic affects the entire body and produces a state of unconsciousness. The purpose of general anaesthesia is to render the patient free of pain. Examples of general anaesthetic solutions are Pentothal and Brebital.

Nitrous oxide is an inhalant type of anaesthesia which produces a semiconscious state. It is occasionally referred to as "laughing gas." It is used with oxygen and produces prompt results and recovery. The use of nitrous oxide is referred to as conscious sedation, and the insurance code is listed in the Adjunctive General section of the dental fee guide.

Antibiotics are chemical substances produced by a microorganism (bacterium, yeast, or mould) that inhibit or stop the growth of bacteria, fungi, or parasites. The prefix *anti* means against, and *bio* means life, which means that the properties of an antibiotic inhibit the growth of bacterial life.

If a patient has a history of heart disease of any kind or joint replacement, the doctor may recommend the prophylactic administration of antibiotics. During every dental surgical procedure, there is a danger of bacterial infection as a result of bleeding.

TABLE 17.1 **ABBREVIATIONS**

LATIN ABBREVIATION	ENGLISH EQUIVALENT
a.a.	of each
a.c.	before meals
AD	right ear
AS	left ear
b.i.d.	twice daily
c	with
caps	capsule
disp	dispense
dtd	give this number
et	and
ext	external use
gtt	drop
hs	hour of sleep (bedtime)
M ft	make
mitt#	give this number
ml	millilitre
OD	right eye, or overdose
OS	left eye
p.c.	after meals
p.o.	by mouth
p.r.n.	as needed
q	every
q.d.	once a day
q.i.d.	four times daily
Sig.	label as follows
sl	under the tongue, sublingual
SOB	shortness of breath
stat	at once, first dose
q.2h	every two hours
Rx	take thou
t.i.d.	three times a day

The most common form of antibiotic that is prescribed is penicillin, which is available in a variety of formulas and sold under many different names. If the patient has a hypersensitive reaction to penicillin, the dentist will recommend an alternative such as Erythromycin, which closely resembles penicillin but does not cause the same adverse reaction.

Although the dental office administrator does not prescribe the medication, patients should be asked if they have ever experienced a reaction to the medication or if they are taking any other medications. You should also ask if they understand how to administer the medication. The use of antibiotics should be continued until the medication is completed. Many patients will stop taking medications when they feel better, and infections may recur.

Antihistamines are drugs that block the action of histamine, which is released during an allergic reaction. In severe cases, the allergic reaction can cause anaphylactic shock. Many of these drugs can contain an anti-emetic (such as Dramamine) to prevent nausea and vomiting. Some examples of antihistamines are Chlor Trimetron and Benadryl.

Vasoconstrictors narrow blood vessels to raise blood pressure and are commonly used in cardiac or respiratory failure. Epinephrine is a vasoconstrictor that stimulates the heart. It has many applications in dentistry, and is also included in small quantities with local anaesthetic solutions.

Vasodilators open or dilate blood vessels to reduce blood pressure and slow the heart beat. Nitroglycerin is a vasodilator and is usually administered below the tongue (sublingually), but it can be administered via a spray or a transdermal patch.

Anticoagulants are drugs that prevent the clotting of blood. They are used to prevent the formation of clots or to break up clots in blood vessels. Heparin is a natural anticoagulant produced in the liver cells. Common types of anticoagulants are Coumadin (sodium warfarin) and dicoumarol. Aspirin, which is prescribed for patients who suffer from arthritis, can produce an effect similar to that of an anticoagulant. It is important for the dentist to know if the patient is taking any type of anticoagulant medication before commencing with a dental procedure. Hemostasis (control of blood flow) is much more difficult on patients who are taking anticoagulants.

Anticonvulsants prevent or reduce the severity of convulsions in various types of epilepsy. Some common anticonvulsive agents are Dilantin (phenytoin), phenobarbital, and Tegretol.

Sedatives are drugs that calm nervousness and anxiety by depressing the central nervous system. These include hypnotics that induce sleep. Drugs that have a calming effect include Atarax, Restoril, Xanax, and Valium.

Stimulants act on the brain to speed up vital processes in cases of shock and collapse. Caffeine is contained in many drugs that constrict the cerebral blood vessels, for example, Dexedrine and Ritalin.

Tranquillizers are useful in controlling anxiety by calming certain areas of the brain, while permitting the rest of the brain to function normally. They act as a screen that allows transmission of some nerve impulses but restricts others. The drug most frequently used is phenothiazine.

Routes of Drug Administration

There are several factors that determine how the drug should be introduced into the body. Medication must be used correctly to produce the full effect and obtain the expected results. Improperly administered drugs can produce dangerous side effects and may even become toxic. The dentist will decide how the drug should be administered and how quickly the desired effect can be achieved.

The side effects of a drug are known as the therapeutic effects or drug activity. An adverse reaction to a drug can cause an undesirable effect that, in some cases, can be lethal.

There are several ways to administer drugs, and how they are administered affects their action.

1. **Oral**—by mouth (p.o.) in the form of a pill, tablet, capsule, or liquid.

    Liquid solutions may be in the form of a saturated solution in which the drug particles are completely dissolved in the solution. A stock solution is one in which the drug is close to saturation point. It is highly concentrated and can be used to make weaker solutions. An oral suspension is a solution in which the drug particles remain in their solid form or stay suspended. This type of solution will be identified with a label that states "shake well."

    The most common form of oral medication is in a solid state such as a pill, tablet, or capsule. Pills and tablets are pressed discs made with a sugar or starch mix to which the drug is added. Many pills have an enteric coating to keep the medication from dissolving as it passes through the stomach. It will dissolve in the intestine and be absorbed into the bloodstream. Capsules are gelatin containers with the powder or liquid form of the drug inside. The gelatin capsule dissolves in the stomach.

The oral route of drug administration is the safest and most economical route; however, it produces a slower response time than other methods.

2. **Sublingual**—under the tongue. This route of administration absorbs the medication through the mucosa of the floor of the mouth. Some drugs are absorbed rapidly in highly concentrated dosages. Nitroglycerin is often administered sublingually.

3. **Inhalant**—by breathing in a gaseous substance. This is one of the fastest routes of absorption and results in no decomposition of the drug. Oral aerosol inhalers are used for asthma and other breathing disorders. The drug is absorbed deep in the lungs where it is most effective. An aerosol contains the drug in a solution which can be inhaled for respiratory problems or sprayed topically on the skin surface. The effect is usually immediate. The most common type of inhalant medication used in dentistry is nitrous oxide.

4. **Rectal**—inserted into the rectum in suppository form. This route can be used on an unconscious or mentally ill patient or when slow absorption through the colon walls is required. It is an alternative when oral administration of a drug is contraindicated. Suppositories are composed of a material which will melt at body temperature. The drug is embedded in the suppository.

5. **Topical**—applied to the surface of the skin or mucous membranes. It is effective for localized absorption but slower than other routes.

6. **Parenteral**—by injection. An injection under the skin is called *subcutaneous* (below the lower layer of skin). Injection into the muscle (IM) is an *intramuscular* injection; into the vein (IV) is an *intravenous* injection, the most rapid route of all.

The parenteral route has the advantage of producing rapid and predictable results and is used for emergencies. It is expensive, requires a certain amount of skill to administer, and may result in infection at the site of the injection.

7. **Transdermal**—through skin patches. Transdermal patches allow controlled, continuous release of medication such as nitroglycerin. They are convenient and easy to use. Skin irritation may occur and it is recommended that the site of application be changed from time to time.

In general, when a drug is absorbed through a body membrane such as the skin, mucosa of the mouth, stomach, or colon, larger doses must be given.

NARCOTICS CONTROL

An accurate and complete record must be kept of each drug that has been prescribed to a patient. Notation must be made on the patient's chart giving information about the prescription and the route of administration. When a drug is administered in the office, it should be recorded on the patient's chart.

A record must be kept of any narcotics that are stored in the office and administered to patients. The dental office administrator should be aware that narcotics cannot be ordered without a written prescription. The dentist's telephone prescription orders should be followed up with a written prescription.

When a pharmacist calls the office, the dentist should be notified immediately. The dentist is the only person who is legally qualified to prescribe and administer medications. If he or she cannot be disturbed, the administrator should take a complete message and give it to the dentist at the first opportunity. Ask the pharmacist to slowly spell the name of the patient and the medication to help with accurate recording of the information.

An accurate inventory of all medications that are stored in the office should be maintained, including samples that have been left by drug company representatives. Every medication that is administered within the office should be accounted for. All medications should be kept in a locked cabinet.

A sign-out sheet should be kept to provide an audit trail for drug administration. Each person must sign and date the sign-out sheet before the medication is dispensed.

TABLE 17.2 MEDICATION SIGN-OUT SHEET

Name of Patient	Medication	Signature/Date
Susan Smith	Tylenol	Jan. 2/96, S. Scaler
John Brown	Motrin, 200 mg 4 tabs	Jan. 3/96, R. Assistant
Dave Dole	Tylenol 3, 50 mg 4 tabs	Jan. 4/96 Dr. Kay

EXHIBIT 17.2 RECORD OF PRESCRIPTION

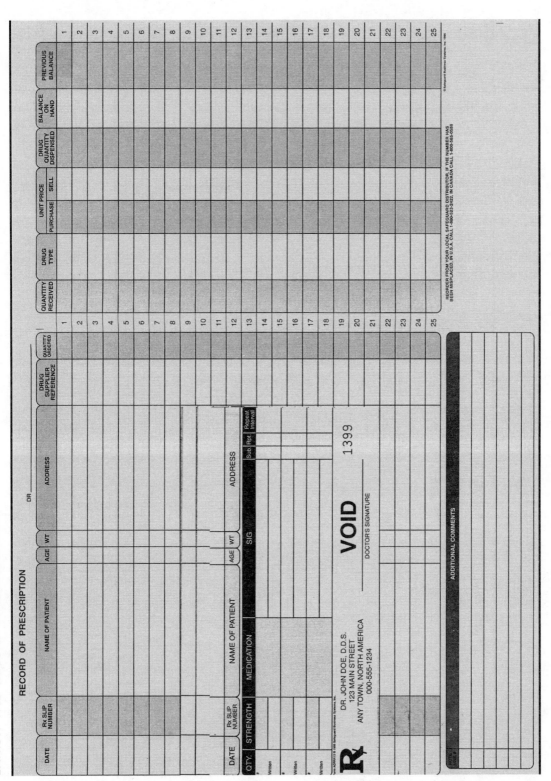

Used with permission by Safeguard Business Systems, Inc., Fort Washington, PA 19034

EXHIBIT 17.3   DRUG INVENTORY LEDGER

DRUG INVENTORY LEDGER

DRUG _____

EXPIRATION DATE _____

BALANCE FORWARD

DATE	Rx SLIP NUMBER	NAME OF PATIENT	AGE	WT	ADDRESS	DRUG SUPPLIER REFERENCE	QUANTITY ORDERED	QUANTITY RECEIVED	DRUG TYPE	UNIT PRICE PURCHASE	UNIT PRICE SELL	DRUG QUANTITY DISPENSED	BALANCE ON HAND	PREVIOUS BALANCE	
															1
															2
															3
															4
															5
															6
															7
															8
															9
															10
															11
															12
															13
															14
															15
															16
															17
															18
															19
															2

Used with permission by Safeguard Business Systems, Inc., Fort Washington, PA 19034

DRUG ACTION

The administrator should never try to evaluate a patient's reaction to a drug. The dentist is the only person who is qualified to do this. The administrator cannot diagnose or evaluate the patient's status. Interrupt the dentist immediately if necessary or have the dentist call the patient back.

When a drug enters the body, the target substance with which the drug interacts is called a receptor. The following terms describe the action and interaction of drugs in the body after they have been absorbed into the bloodstream.

Additive Action—The combination of two similar drugs is equal to the sum of the effects of each. For example, if one drug has a 10 percent effect and another has 20 percent effect, the combination of both will create a 30 percent effect.

Cumulative Action—After administration of certain drugs, concentrations of them or their toxic effect may increase with each dose. Some drugs are not quickly eliminated from the body.

Idiosyncrasy—This is an unexpected or peculiar reaction that may appear in the patient following administration of a drug.

Synergism—When two drugs are combined, the effect is greater than if they were given alone. For example, penicillin and streptomycin are given together in treatment of bacterial endocarditis because of their synergistic properties.

Tolerance—A patient withstands the normal dose and the effects diminish as treatment goes on. Larger doses must be given to maintain the desired effect. This is a feature of addiction to drugs such as morphine or Demerol.

Antagonism—Drugs that are combined have an undesirable effect.

Hypersensitivity—The body will produce antibodies for protection. A hypersensitive reaction is an exaggerated immune response.

Intolerance —This is a reaction greater than expected from a normal or small dose.

Side Effect —An unavoidable effect may result from taking an average dose of a drug.

Addiction—This is excessive and continued use of habit-forming drugs. A person who physically depends on a drug builds a tolerance to it and requires larger doses. A withdrawal state is experienced when the drug is stopped.

Habituation—A patient may, over time, develop a psychological desire to keep using a drug.

Drug abuse—Abuse can involve misuse of prescription or illegal drugs.

Overdose—An undesirable effect results from taking too much of a drug. A toxic overdose causes poisoning and a lethal overdose will cause death.

Antidote—This is a substance used to neutralize or lessen the toxicity of a poison.

MEDICATIONS MANAGEMENT

Medical preparations are of value only if they retain their therapeutic activity and identity. Exposure to air, light, moisture, and temperature changes can affect their quality and effectiveness. A basic policy for the storage of medications and materials is to keep them in a dry, cool place where they are not exposed to direct sunlight. Caution should always be taken to note the expiration date that may be listed on medications.

The dental office administrator should always be aware of and comply with drug control regulations. Be alert to the possibility of someone trying to steal drugs from the office. Narcotics must be kept in a locked cabinet and drug samples kept out of sight and reach. Prescription pads should be kept in locked storage. The administrator should be alert to the possibility of someone trying to forge or alter a prescription. The dentist should be told if there is suspicion of anyone doing this.

Used disposable syringes and needles should be broken and disposed of properly. Drugs and drug samples should not be abused by the staff or used for self-medication.

The dental office administrator should never give a patient any medication. Dispensing of drugs without explicit written instructions from the dentist or a doctor is a violation of the law.

PREMEDICATION PROCEDURES

Premedication is medication given in advance of treatment. It may be administered to relieve the anxiety of an apprehensive patient. Many dentists will premedicate patients with prophylactic antibiotics. These are usually prescribed as a preventive measure for patients who have a known history of cardiac problems. The heart is the central pump of the circulatory system and is susceptible to bacterial endocarditis.

Endocarditis is infection of the endocardium, or inner lining of the heart, and the heart valves which control the movement of blood through the heart. When bleeding occurs during a dental procedure, bacteria from the mouth enter the bloodstream. The bacteria invade the valves and produce vegetative growth. Endocarditis can cause severe valvular damage, which can lead to insufficiency and congestive heart failure. If left untreated, endocarditis is usually fatal. However, with proper treatment, approximately 70 percent of patients recover.

As a precaution, the dentist may prescribe high doses of antibiotics to be taken prior to the dental appointment. Some dentists prefer that the patient start taking antibiotics 24 hours in advance of the appointment, while others feel that a larger dose one to two hours in advance is adequate.

The dental office administrator should discuss the premedication policy with the dentist and record step by step procedures on file cards for easy access and quick reference.

General procedures for premedication are as follows:

1. As the charts are being pulled for the next day, each one should be checked for medical alert status. This will be indicated somewhere on the chart in red.

2. Call the patient to confirm the appointment and verify whether he or she has begun the medication or needs to have a prescription called in to the pharmacy. It is illegal for a dental office administrator to call in a prescription for a narcotic; however, antibiotic prescriptions can be called in as a courtesy to the patient.

EXHIBIT 17.4 PREMEDICATION PROCEDURES

Call the pharmacy. (Shoppers Drugs 555-2345—Bill is the pharmacist.)
Identify yourself and the office, ask to speak to the pharmacist to call in a prescription.
If it is a prescription renewal, identify it as such.
Normal dosages: Pen VK 350 mg, 24 tabs, Erythromycin 200 mg, etc.
Record in red in the patient's chart, including the date and time.
Instruct the patient regarding pick-up and administration of prescription.

3. Ask the patient if there has been any change in medical status or allergies.
4. Ask the patient the name of the pharmacy preferred and telephone number if possible. Tell the patient that you will order the medication from the pharmacy, to be picked up at his or her convenience. Remind the patient that the medication is necessary for his or her own protection.
5. Call the pharmacy. Ask to speak to the pharmacist. Identify the office and the purpose of your call. There may be a great deal of background noise at the pharmacy. Speak clearly to ensure the accuracy of the message.
6. Record the information accurately on the patient's chart. Underline the information in red to draw the attention of the dentist.

Many patients appreciate a reminder that they require a prescription before their dental appointment. Failure to follow appropriate premedication procedures may expose the patient to an unnecessary and preventable health risk. In addition, the dentist is also exposed to the risk of legal action.

ASSIGNMENT

1. On the prescription provided below, indicate the components of a prescription. Read the prescription as if you were telling a patient what the drug is, how much to take and when, and whether there are refills.
2. Do some research to determine what the main ingredient of the drug is, its use, any side effects, and what the dentist should be aware of when prescribing this medication.
3. What side effects can this drug cause?
4. What additional advice would you give the patient?

Dr. D. Kay

123 Cuspid Court

Winnipeg, Manitoba, M8J 9K9

Reg. # 394857676398404-87

Name of Patient:_____   Age _____

Address:_____

Rx

PenVee 350 mg

24 capsules

Sig: 1 caps q4h, p.r.n. e.t. h.s.

Refill 2×   _____

CHAPTER EIGHTEEN

MARKETING THE DENTAL PRACTICE

OBJECTIVE

At the end of this chapter, the student will be able to identify and describe the following: a marketing strategy, the role of the dental office administrator in point-of-sale marketing, and specific marketing ideas.

TOPICS

- definition of marketing
- role of the dental team in marketing strategy
- business strategies
- informed choices
- marketing strategy
- client trust
- suggested marketing techniques

WHAT IS MARKETING?

Marketing is vital to all economic growth and development. It is a system of activities to identify and satisfy consumer needs and wants. In primitive economies, markets were traditionally held at an open square in the centre of a town. Products and services would be displayed and sold at these markets. The fundamentals of marketing are product, place, price, and promotion. One must also understand the concept of supply and demand and have a plan of action.

The process of selling products and services can be slow and cumbersome. The producers or providers of the service are not always the most qualified to sell them. Markets need "merchants" to facilitate the exchange of goods and services. These merchants or salespeople have come to be known as wholesalers and retailers in product marketing. The world of trade and economic activity is based on this concept. In dentistry, the dental team members are the marketing facilitators or merchants. When the team performs the function of market facilitators, this allows the dentist to concentrate on providing the best possible dental care to the patients, who are the consumers.

Until recent years, Canadian dentists have been severely restricted in how they were allowed to advertise. Advertising restrictions were probably imposed to help maintain control of professional conduct and the ethical responsibilities associated with health care delivery. Such restrictions provide guidelines that are congruent with the philosophy of the Health Disciplines Act in Canada. How, then, do dentists announce to the public that they have a service of value to sell? The answer is through the implementation of effective marketing techniques.

Product and Price

The challenge faced by dental professionals is to announce to the public that they have a service to sell which is of value to the dental consumer. The consumer must be assured of receiving quality care and value for the money. In general, most people are willing to spend a few extra dollars if they feel that a service is of value to them.

The public is made up of informed consumers who do not want to be misled by gimmicky advertising. The Canadian consumer has become increasingly health conscious in recent years and, because dentistry is a health care service, dental office administrators should meet the needs of the consumer by providing information. Information allows the Canadian consumer to make informed choices.

A dental patient will very seldom select a service based on the price alone. Price is just one of many factors that the consumer will consider.

Price does not assure the patient that he or she will be receiving the most appropriate treatment. Overemphasis on price and discounted fees based on insurance plans promote a perception of discount dentistry and damage every aspect of the profession that relates to the quality of health care delivery.

Location

Visibility and accessibility are two very important considerations that should be taken into account when the practice is established. The office should be easily found in a highly visible location. Adequate and accessible parking are necessary to encourage repeat business. Accessibility for disabled patients is absolutely essential.

It is important to understand the fundamental characteristics of the community that will be serviced, such as the demographics and population, in order to understand how the marketing program should be targeted. For example, new home developments usually have a large number of young families. The target market would be parents of young children. More established neighbourhoods may project different consumer needs, such as a focus on adult preventive dental care.

Specific target marketing begins with sensitivity to the needs and wants of the patient. Knowing what is of value to your patients and understanding their demographic and psychological considerations are essential to achieve patient loyalty and commitment, promote repeat business, and create new business.

INFORMED CHOICES

When patients feel comfortable they are more likely to return for treatment, refer friends, and keep their appointments. The process begins with the creation of a new experience at the time of each visit to the dental office. The dental office administrator should assume the role of relationship coordinator, ensuring that every patient leaves the office with a secure feeling of knowing that he or she has received quality treatment. Marketing will not work unless there is sincerity and caring behind it, which is reflected in the attitude of the team. The patients make the treatment choices and should be gently guided by the dental team to make informed, intelligent ones.

It is the job of the merchant to gently guide the patient toward selecting the optimal treatment by making it as attractive as possible. For example, consider for a moment a consumer who is planning to change hairstyles. Which hairdresser would be more attractive?

"Cheap Cuts R Us"

"Expert Hair Sculpting and Design"

If consumers are willing to pay more for what they perceive to be a superior quality of service, how would they determine if the service is superior? Does the title affect the quality of the service? How is the perceived quality of the service or product affected by the location, visibility, and price?

Consumers are careful and well informed. The majority have less disposable income in today's economic climate than previously. This means that more careful choices must be made and more are value based choices. People now prioritize their needs and budget for goods and services that are of value to them.

THE ROLE OF THE DENTAL TEAM IN MARKETING STRATEGY

A healthy growing relationship between the dentist and the dental team is an important aspect in marketing. The most important marketing tool in a service industry, such as dentistry, is the office personnel.

The new patient experience in a dental office is a critical process in establishing trust and loyalty. Management must be patient-conscious at all times and expect the dental team to exhibit the same behaviour. Revolving staff means revolving patients; high staff turnover is very costly to the practice. Productivity through people is the root of profitability. Dental team members must understand what makes their service work and be keenly motivated.

Enthusiastic dental team members can be effective marketing facilitators by reinforcing treatment and encouraging patient loyalty to the practice. They promote patient referrals and offer creative ideas for newsletters, office brochures, etc. Hygiene staff provide counselling services regarding nutrition and oral health. In effect, they become wellness specialists, providing positive reinforcement for health and reassuring the dental patient that health is a worthwhile investment.

The dental office administrator is the binding force that joins the clinical aspects of dentistry to the business of dentistry. You become the relationship coordinator and merchant by helping the patient to understand the treatment, the necessity for follow-up, and the costs of treatment. You essentially encourage the patient to participate in the overall process of dental treatment. You are also responsible for establishing and maintaining fair but firm financial policies so that the patient knows what to expect and is willing to cooperate.

The marketing plan should be supported by everyone on the dental team. They should be aware of the overhead costs and productivity needed to sustain the practice as well as the requirements of the patients.

One dental receptionist justified the fact that she neglected to perform follow-up and recare calls by stating: "Well, people just don't have the money nowadays, do they? Everyone is being laid off and they do not have dental insurance any more."

This particular receptionist projected her own values onto the patients. She believed that a patient's choice of treatment was based on the availability of insurance coverage. She also assumed that with no dental plan, patients would not value treatment. She prejudged the patients' ability to pay and their willingness to purchase a valuable service. The consequences of her actions were that the entire practice suffered immeasurable financial loss during her term of employment at that office.

Dental insurance and financial considerations are always foremost in the decision-making process of the patient. A dental office administrator should never judge a patient's ability to pay and never presume to know his or her value system. The value system of each individual will determine the acceptance of treatment. The dental office administrator must be careful not to judge people in any way, especially when it comes to paying a bill. Others' value systems may differ from yours because their life circumstances differ.

To demonstrate this point, you could research the marketplace. This would involve measuring the perceptions of dental patients to determine what is of value to them. A sample inquiry might be

> If you had $100 to spend on your appearance, how would you spend it? Which would you value more, a $100 investment in hair care or clothing or $100 worth of dental care?

When patients comment that fees are too high, they may simply mean that they do not choose to buy the service. They may be afraid that it will hurt, or concerned that the dentist will be putting them in a vulnerable position and violating their intimate zone. Consumer lethargy is another cause. In other words, if it is not a life or death health care matter, it can wait.

PATIENT/PROVIDER TRUST

The dental team should be close to the patient, to listen with intent and without judgment to determine what his or her needs are. It is important to respect the patient's point of view at all times. Barriers to communication can be eliminated when the patient feels understood, listened to, and respected.

During the initial interview or new patient experience, the dental office administrator should ask probing questions that will elicit the patient's trust. Probing questions consist of open-ended questions (who, what, where, when, why, how) to draw information. Active listening and paraphrasing helps the patient to feel that he or she is being understood. Direct eye contact and open gestures are essential to gain trust. Once a high trust and low fear relationship exists, it is easier to discover what the individual needs of the patient are and then together develop a treatment program that is congruent with the patient's values. Differing patient needs will reflect different relationships.

1. *Emergency relationship.* A patient may want only this type of relationship. If so, note it somewhere on the chart and don't try to market preventive care.
2. *Restorative or remedial relationship.* Allow room for trust and gently guide the patient toward optimal choice of treatment.
3. *Self-care relationship.* All patients should be encouraged to develop an ongoing maintenance relationship. This is the basis for preventive health care.
4. *Systems relationship.* Proper dental function affects other body systems. This is the total wellness relationship, and the dental team members are the wellness specialists.

THE MARKETING PLAN

The word *strategy* means to lead. A business strategy is a careful plan or method for achieving a desired result. You must identify a specific marketing objective in order to develop a strategy to get there. It is similar to using a road map to arrive at a specified destination. Participants can help their roles, and visualize and discuss the expected result.

The dental office administrator should monitor the progress of the marketing program to determine how many new patients selected the office as a direct result. This helps to measure the growth of the practice and to project future growth trends.

Each dental office should develop a marketing budget. Once the budget is established, it is important to determine how the dollars would best be spent to appeal to the target market. New and unique approaches to marketing can involve all of the dental service providers through sharing ideas and careful planning. Provincial dental association guidelines regarding marketing and advertising should be complied with at all times.

Planning the marketing strategy includes periodically taking the time to list the problems encountered and prioritize any necessary changes for the future. Review the plan's progress and identify barriers encountered in order to redirect the marketing focus if necessary. Included with the marketing strategy should be some type of reward for the dental team members for their involvement and support. Positive reinforcement encourages repeated positive behaviour.

Electronic Marketing

Computers in dental offices enhance internal marketing programs by providing ongoing support and organizational management functions. They will store and sort statistical information, which aids marketing tasks, such as recalls, treatment plan follow-ups, predetermination items, birthdates, and special occasions. A word processing package will produce newsletters, personal letters, thank-you letters, formal reports, manuscripts for publication, and transcriptions of dental records.

Intra-oral computers allow the dentist to see problems that are not always evident to the naked eye and not visible on x-rays. These are valuable educational tools that assist the patient with understanding the treatment by providing before and after pictures.

The marketing of dental services may be considered as more than just a means to a profitable business. It can be viewed as a community service that promotes preventive health care. Wellness promotion can reduce the overall costs of health care to the public. This means that the cost of dental insurance plans could substantially decrease to be more affordable and available to a larger portion of the population.

Community outreach to promote dental health education is an effective method of marketing dental services that remains within ethical guidelines. For example, during Dental Health Week, some offices will invite parents to bring in their children who are athletically inclined to have a sports guard made free of charge. If even one or two new families decide to continue to be treated at the office, the cost of running the clinic will be well worth it.

If the target market consists of families with small children, mothers may be invited to bring in preschoolers to visit the office. To reach this market segment, administrators of local preschools, daycare centres or kindergartens could be contacted. The children could be invited to visit the office and learn about preventive dental care, such as toothbrushing and eating healthy foods. As the children leave, they could be provided with information packages about the office that include a toothbrush and the name and address of the office.

Specific Marketing Ideas

The marketing presentation should enhance the office image and confirm the values of the dental team. The following are some specific suggestions:

- Incorporate **symbolism** into the office image. A bright red apple can symbolize health and complement your image as a wellness resource.
- Hand out a **pocket toothbrush** with the dentist's name and phone number printed on it.
- Send **letters directly to kids;** they love to receive mail.
- Do not send the same recall cards all the time. Choose **card designs** that will attract the attention of your target market.
- Send a **newsletter** to all of your patients. Involve the staff in its creation. Provide news information related to dentistry—for example, infection control procedures, mercury contamination, x-ray safety, new dental procedures, etc. Nutritional information including sugar-free recipes can be provided by the hygiene team, and a kids' corner will make it of interest to children.
- Hold a **monthly draw for a CD or video** for the children and teens in your practice. Announce the winner in the newsletter.
- A **frequent referral program** is an incentive for patients to refer their friends and relatives. Perhaps after five new people have selected your practice through their referral, patients could win a dinner for two at a local restaurant.
- A **special occasion prophylaxis** could be the reward when a patient refers two new patients. Wouldn't it be nice to have your teeth polished for that special evening, party, or wedding?
- The **smile makeover** can be part of a new look people are searching for by having their hair done, buying a new outfit, etc. Health clubs have capitalized on this concept by opening facilities all over the country. We are a visual society and nothing could be more physically appealing than an attractive, clean, healthy mouth. Perhaps the dental office could offer a free consultation on cosmetic dentistry.

- The **No Cavity Club** is used by most dental offices across the country, where a bulletin board holds Polaroid pictures of children who have had a positive dental visit. Children enjoy looking for their own picture and for pictures of their friends at each visit.
- **Flowers on Mother's Day** add a cheerful note to the dental office. Have fresh carnations or roses at the front counter and present one to each mother on this special day.
- **Flowers on Father's Day?** Why not?
- On **Halloween**, have all of the staff dress up, and ask your patients to vote on the best costume. Encourage all of the children to visit your practice that day and have someone available to distribute sugar-free gum and/or toothbrushes printed with the name of the office and telephone number.
- Send **birthday cards** signed by the staff to all patients. A computerized reminder system will be helpful for this. (See Exhibit 18.1 for an example.)
- On a **Good News Bulletin Board**, display good news items about patients—for example, Mrs. Smith had a baby girl. Be sure to obtain the patient's permission first.
- Invite patients to snip out **recipes** from magazines while they are waiting, using safety scissors left in the reception area.
- **Fridge magnets** provide a constant reminder of your dental office.
- **Information brochures** can publicize the name and address of the office.

Continuing Education and the Dental Team

Consumers of dental services should be informed that the dental service providers continue to increase their knowledge and skills through continuing education. Emphasis on this will reassure patients that they are receiving the most up-to-date dental care possible. Technology, materials, and procedures change at such a rapid pace that it is critical for dental team members to remain current. Many of the provincial dental assistant and hygiene associations require their members to continuously upgrade their education in order to maintain their certification status. In some provinces, certification of dental office administrators is encouraged. Continuing education enhances the professional image of the office, increases motivation and enthusiasm, and cultivates professional integrity.

EXHIBIT 18.1 COMPUTER-GENERATED BIRTHDAY LIST

Birthdays

Printed: 03/MAR/.95 06:11p
Page 1   Accounting Date: 03/MAR/95

Patient ID	Birthdate	Full Name	Sex	Phone No.	Age
06391	12/MAR/89	CARMON, Emily J. 5443 Sunny St. Burlington, Ontario L0H 2H0	F	(905)343–5028 (905)684–5800	5
00250	13/MAR/87	DENINGER, Harry J. 45 Nice St. Hamilton, Ontario L7N 1W5	M	(905)755–3439 (905)743–0000	7
10621	09/MAR/90	GARRET, Joe Box 440, R.R. #3 Caledonia, Ontario L0H 1G0	M	(905)432–5178 (905)343–8756	4
09439	10/MAR/90	HUSTON, Anna 651 Pembridge Cres. Caledonia, Ontario L0H 2G3	F	(905)434–3761 (905)343–4230	4
04643	09/MAR/87	JONES, Leslie E. Box 55, R.R. #1 Caledonia, Ontario L0H 1G0	F	(905)433–3167 (905)433–3000	
10644	12/MAR/87	SILVER, Sidney 1079 Main St. Burlington, Ontario L7P 2S3	M	(905)389–0401 (905)356–7882	7
08622	10/MAR/88	THOMAS, Barry 109 York Street Hamilton, Ontario L7K 1P9	F	(905)567–8215 (905)959-4400	6

Sample provided by ABEL Computers Ltd., Burlington, Ontario.

ASSIGNMENT

1. Conduct some market research by completing the following patient survey. Determine how your friends and neighbours feel about their dental treatment. Measure the general perceptions of dental office patients and try to determine what is of value to the market that you surveyed. Write three to four paragraphs discussing your observations. Submit the assignment to your instructor. Discuss findings with the class.
2. Define *marketing strategy.*
3. What factors would cause changes in marketing strategy?
4. Create a marketing strategy for a fictitious dental office. Create the demographics of the community and define the needs of the study group.

DENTAL PATIENT SURVEY

Please take a moment to complete the following questionnaire. Record the number in the right hand column that most accurately reflects your answer.

1 = Yes
2 = Usually
3 = Do Not Know
4 = Not Usually
5 = No

	1	2	3	4	5
1. When I telephone my dentist's office, I receive prompt, courteous attention.	—	—	—	—	—
2. All members of the dental team are friendly and courteous.	—	—	—	—	—
3. The dentist listens to me.	—	—	—	—	—
4. The dentist spends enough time with me	—	—	—	—	—
5. The dentist speaks to me in terms that I can understand.	—	—	—	—	—
6. The dentist remembers something about me from visit to visit.	—	—	—	—	—
7. The dentist and staff dress and act professionally.	—	—	—	—	—
8. The dentist and staff help me feel comfortable regarding treatment.	—	—	—	—	—
9. The dental office is clean and well organized.	—	—	—	—	—
10. The reception area is comfortable.	—	—	—	—	—
11. The dental office is conveniently located.	—	—	—	—	—
12. When the dental staff collect personal information, they are respectful of my right to privacy.	—	—	—	—	—
13. The dentist discusses fees and treatment procedures with me before beginning treatment.	—	—	—	—	—
14. The dental staff are competent.	—	—	—	—	—
15. I have learned a lot about taking care of my teeth from the dental staff.	—	—	—	—	—

16. I visit the dentist
__ every six months __ every nine months __ every year
__ more frequently than six months __ less frequently than every year

17. The things I like the most about my dentist are

_____

18. I am happy to refer friends and relatives to my dentist Y_____ N_____

CHAPTER NINETEEN

PERSONNEL RELATIONS

OBJECTIVE

At the end of this chapter, the student will be able to identify and describe the following: the difference between coordinating a group of professionals and managing staff, how to establish and maintain an office policy, team-building skills, problem-solving skills, hiring, firing, and how to conduct team meetings.

TOPICS

- coordinating staff versus managing
- hiring the right team
- establishing office policy
- effective team building
- delegating responsibilities
- problem solving techniques

OFFICE MANAGEMENT

A business manager is one who directs an enterprise and is skilled in managing business affairs. The dental office administrator performs many management duties including personnel management. One of the main responsibilities of the administrator is to create and maintain a harmonious workplace, while facilitating a highly productive and financially viable business. Dental professionals who work together as a team toward a common goal need a leader or activity coordinator to help them achieve their goals. The term "manager" has become somewhat obsolete and is often replaced with "office coordinator" or "team leader." An effective leader is one who displays initiative and caring and enthusiastically accepts new challenges.

Hiring the Right Team Member

Staff turnover is costly for the dentist. Although the estimated cost to replace even one staff member can vary, the time spent screening applicants and interviewing, lost production time, and the dentist's time contribute to the high cost of the hiring. When the dentist is not practising dentistry, income is not being generated; therefore, it is lost income. Hiring the right staff member in the first place can save a tremendous amount of time, energy, and money.

Many dental professionals have had very little training in labour relations and human resources management. In fact, a smaller allotment of education time for Canadian dentists is devoted to practice administration than in the United States. To compensate for this, many dentists will seek the assistance of a skilled business manager/coordinator or consultants who specialize in the field of human relations. A motivated dental office administrator can become the human resource specialist.

Wrongful Hiring

Wrongful hiring can result in staff disruption and have a devastating impact on the morale and motivation of staff members. In addition, the dentist can be exposed to the risk of legal action if proper hiring and firing procedures are not followed.

It is important to know that promises made during an interview can constitute a contract enforceable by law. If promises are not kept, there may be successful claims against the employer stating misrepresentation. If an employer, for example, misrepresents significant aspects of the job during an interview, such as assurances of higher income or improved opportunities, and causes an employee to leave a previous secure job, the employee can sue for damages. It must be proved, however, that the statements were made with intentional negligence.

Some dental professionals will delegate the responsibility of hiring to a placement service which will screen the applicants and their résumés, arrange interviews, and provide reference checks.

Wrongful Dismissal

An employer can be held liable for wrongful dismissal if proper procedures are not carried out for the termination of employees. The first 90 days of employment are usually considered to be a probationary period, during which, if an employer wishes to terminate an employee without notice, he or she can do so without consequence. When an employee has been working for a longer period of time, an employer must provide the employee with the opportunity to improve the behaviour in question.

The first warning can be oral. A second warning to an employee should be in written form and presented to the employee to sign for verification of the warning. Most often, when the warning reaches this particular stage, the employee will quit. It is recommended that an impartial witness be present during these warnings as further protection for both parties. The employee can then be terminated.

At the time of termination an employee must be paid all outstanding holiday pay which has accumulated, along with the final paycheque. As a courtesy, many employers will include severance pay in lieu of notice. This is given as a courtesy only and is not mandatory on termination. It is wise to escort the terminated employee out of the building.

Employers should carefully assess their hiring needs before recruiting new employees. Employers can protect themselves by providing written job descriptions and creating a script to follow during the interview. The job description should resemble the job itself.

Guidelines to Hiring

- Define the office environment. Determine what the office image is and how the current employees reflect that image.
- Analyze the team dynamics. Find out what makes the team work and what does not. Select an overall set of characteristics that would indicate the type of employee who would work in harmony with the team.
- Identify who would *not* fit well with the team. Hiring the wrong person can cause disruption and discord and create a negative working environment. These problems can be prevented by being a proactive office manager/coordinator as opposed to a reactive one.

- Set clear objectives. Decide what skills are important and how much experience is necessary.
- Ask probing questions to determine what the employment candidate can contribute to the dental practice and if he or she is prepared to offer a strong contribution. If an employee is working only for a paycheque, then he or she clearly lacks motivation and initiative. A motivated employee will have a sense of ownership for the position and display enthusiasm about the work.
- Establish a set of questions that meet the established objective. Ask open ended questions which will encourage the candidate to elaborate. Open-ended questions are those that begin with the five "W's" (who, what, where, when, why) or how.

During the interview, observe the body language of the potential employee. Body language does not lie. Eye contact is important as it displays sincerity and honesty. Look for an employee who displays positive nonverbal communications. A smile, for example, is one of the most powerful nonverbal forms of communication. A confident employment candidate with a positive attitude will display open gestures and friendly mannerisms. Good manners also create a positive first impression.

Observe how the candidate is dressed. Most dental offices maintain a policy of proper dress. Although the interviewer's interest is also directed to work performance and human relations ability, personal appearance and grooming standards represent observable behaviour.

It is very difficult to follow up with employees with unacceptable attire after they have been hired. Everyone has a right to express individuality, but an employer should seek an employee who feels that a little conformity won't hurt. This may be a good indication that the employee will be cooperative in other matters also.

Dentistry is a health care profession, so the candidate should also reflect an image of good health and a positive outlook. In addition, the job interview is an opportunity for the employment candidate to display communication skills including appropriate grammatical usage, part of a professional and polished image.

Always check the employee's references. This point cannot be overemphasized. When this step is overlooked, it can lead to serious problems later on and expose the dentist to unnecessary and preventable legal risk.

Résumés

If there is a spelling error on the résumé or cover letter then it is not usually worth considering. Remember that this is an opportunity for the employment candidate to put his or her best foot forward and to reveal information about him or herself that demonstrates a professional tone.

A candidate who has experienced too many job or career changes may have been jumping around from job to job. Candidates with such a history may leave as soon as things do not go their way, or they may be using this employment opportunity as a stepping stone on the road to their true career goal.

Watch for inconsistencies, particularly with dates. If there are large gaps in the employment history, ask why. If the employment candidate refuses to provide references, ask why.

OFFICE PHILOSOPHY

All members of the dental team should understand and believe in the office philosophy or mission statement. If the office does not have a philosophy, then perhaps this could be discussed at a staff meeting. Creating an office philosophy together is an effective team building technique. For example, does your office believe in the importance of preventive dentistry? A positive office image is created and maintained when all members of the dental team are communicating with the patients in a way that is congruent with the office philosophy or mission statement. The mission statement will identify how the dental professionals feel about patient care and provide a vision of personal growth and development for each team member.

Office Policies

The office policies and/or procedures manual represents a clear set of guidelines that establishes specific job objectives and performance expectations and defines specific procedural directives. An effective method of establishing office policies is to negotiate and agree upon them collectively, as a team. This process helps to pre-empt any misunderstandings and clarify the objectives. A fair and well-defined office policy may eliminate conflicts that arise among team members.

An office policy should delineate the duties and responsibilities of each staff member and clarify issues such as vacations, statutory holidays, the dentist's holiday, staff remuneration, sick days, etc.

THE STAFF MEETING

Regularly scheduled staff meetings provide an opportunity to review office philosophy, redefine goals, and decide on the process to achieve goals. They provide an opportunity to share ideas that enhance the growth of the practice. Marketing ideas and strategies can be established through brainstorming sessions. Marketing plans can be very effective when they have full support of the dental team.

Staff meetings are also an opportunity to resolve issues which can grow into conflicts. When issues remain unresolved, tension is created which leads to a build-up of emotionally based issues. Conflict cannot be resolved when it is clouded by emotion. It is much easier to resolve issues as they arise. This helps to prevent hurt feelings and needless dissension.

The staff meeting is also an opportunity to review emergency protocol and identify where emergency equipment is located. Remaining calm in the event of an office emergency is important, and contingency plans can be executed well if all staff know what is expected and conduct themselves in a calm, controlled manner.

Staff meetings are also an opportunity to motivate staff and encourage excellence in service and skill. Providing staff members with positive reinforcement for a job well done will encourage the repetition of positive behaviour and result in employee job satisfaction and a pleasant atmosphere.

The reasons for staff meetings will vary from office to office and the length of the meetings will change according to the needs of the staff. Meetings should be held when income cannot be generated, perhaps over a lunch hour or after normal working hours. An agenda should be used, which may include protocol for the meeting, and a copy should be given to each staff member before the meeting. The agenda should include time for discussion and for all staff members to share their thoughts and suggestions.

One objective that should be considered when organizing staff meetings is to provide each staff member with an opportunity to have his or her voice heard. A nonthreatening atmosphere that promotes openness should be encouraged. A team of dedicated professionals will rely on colleagues as a resource for creativity and problem solving.

The Morning Meeting

Some dentists like to conduct a mini-meeting each morning before the day commences. The morning meeting allows the staff to set the structure for the day. It is essential that all staff members attend the morning session (which can range from 10 to 15 minutes) and that everyone arrives on time.

The purposes of the morning mini-meeting are

- to be prepared for the day, mentally and physically
- to ensure that laboratory work has been received
- to determine where to accommodate emergencies in the schedule
- to identify new patients
- to personalize the schedule and identify patients with special needs
- to provide feedback from the previous day and discuss problems or happy events
- to make general announcements
- to promote communication and lift the morale of all staff at the same time
- to identify the postoperative calls that should be made by the clinical assistant or administrator
- to identify medical alerts—anything that will be significant to the day's treatment
- to identify open appointments (if any) and work toward filling them
- to discuss positive feedback from patients
- to leave with the latest joke or a positive comment to help set the tone for the day

To encourage all staff members to be on time, create an incentive. If they are late for the meeting, request that they donate $2 to the staff fund, which can be used to purchase birthday cakes on staff birthdays or occasional lunches.

DELEGATION OF DUTIES

Delegating job responsibilities and then allowing employees the freedom to perform the given tasks can be difficult. It is often difficult for the dentist or office manager to "let go" and trust employees to do their job. You should provide them with the necessary instructions and safety precautions and then allow them to do it. Do not supervise excessively or hover over them to make sure that the job is done correctly, as this can be degrading and demoralizing to professionals.

Successful delegation will be achieved when the dentist or office manager clearly defines the objective, tells employees what is expected of them and when, and then trusts them to be able to follow instructions. If an employee cannot follow the guidelines that have been provided, then there is clearly a breakdown in the hiring process and perhaps that employee is not suited for the job.

A good office manager or employer will seek to hire winners. They will look for employees who can do the job well and fit in with the existing team. A professional dental office administrator will not feel threatened by this process and will provide all of the team members with a nurturing and rewarding work environment.

ROLE MODEL

Our personal behaviour forms the basis on which we are judged by others. In dentistry, patients often form opinions about the dentist's clinical skills based on many factors, one of which is the behaviour of the dental team. Each member of the dental team becomes a reflection of the office image. It is important, therefore, to be a positive role model to enhance the professional image of the dental practice.

Behaviour is observed and sets an example for others. If a dental employee complains frequently about his or her job or personal life, the dental practice, or anything that is perceived as negative, then other team members will avoid contact with this person as much as possible. The office administrator must be a positive role model and exhibit a happy and optimistic attitude toward him or herself and others.

Be supportive and speak well of those you work with. Avoid office gossip at all costs and set the example for other team members that gossip is not acceptable behaviour. Remember that the principles of confidentiality apply to all aspects of the dental profession. Do not release confidential information and do not engage in conversations that include destructive criticisms of other team members.

When the dental office administrator speaks well of the dental team, it creates a sense of trust and is a positive reflection on their professionalism. Dental professionals should always take pride in their career and the people they work with.

Dentistry is a health care profession and one's dress, mannerisms, and health should reflect a high standard of professionalism. Dental patients expect to see a well-groomed and healthy office administrator. This helps to establish a level of trust with the dental client by showing that the dental team members practise what they preach.

PROBLEM SOLVING

A proactive management philosophy is similar to a preventive dentistry program. A continuous program of dental prevention techniques can prevent minor problems from becoming larger, more painful, and more costly. Proactive management, rather than reactive management, can provide the same positive results.

Small daily irritations and grudges held can be barriers to communication and cause conflicts within the office. If left unresolved, they can accelerate and become damaging. Restoring a working relationship is then more difficult and the conflict can become severe. It may be necessary to seek an intermediary or counsellor to help resolve the conflict. The sooner that the restoration process begins after a relationship has been damaged, the better.

Feelings of frustration or anxiety can temporarily block goals. Frustration almost always causes some form of aggression, whether it is overt or passive aggression. For example, silence can be a form of passive aggressive behaviour. A mature and healthy person will seek acceptable methods for releasing frustrations. It may be through talking with a friend, doing something creative, or going for a walk.

Frustrations occur in every aspect of our lives and our success depends on how well we learn to cope with them. We need to learn to live with frustrations and not allow them to victimize ourselves or others. Recognizing the frustration and analyzing its cause is the first step toward releasing it.

It is important to recognize that the aggressive behaviour of others is also a result of frustration. The dental office administrator needs to be sensitive to the frustrations of others and what their emotional needs are at that moment. Diplomacy and sincere caring will help to resolve conflicts and promote a mature approach to conflict resolution.

Communication is the lifeblood of any relationship and opening the channels of communication is a vital process. To remove the feeling of fear in the communication process, it is important to see the connection between repairing and nurturing relationships and career success.

Be willing to rebuild and repair a damaged relationship. Do not harbour resentment and hold a grudge. Design a rebuilding strategy. Be a good listener—the most difficult part of any human communication is listening. Try to empathize and truly understand what the other person is experiencing.

Inject humour into your communications as much as possible. Humour, when used appropriately, is a great icebreaker. Be sure to use appropriate humour and refrain from derogatory remarks that can be offensive to others, particularly if they are prejudicial in nature.

Give as much to the communication process as you expect to receive. Learn how to swallow your pride and not be afraid to apologize when it is necessary and appropriate. Do not blame; accept responsibility for the breakdown in communication. Demonstrate a healthy and mature attitude by not placing blame on other people or situations that cause you frustration. Learn how to forgive. Be accessible and have an open mind.

STAFF INCENTIVES

Financial remuneration is not the only factor that motivates staff members to contribute to the overall success of the practice. It is, however, the most basic incentive. Experienced dental professionals seek high quality staff members and acknowledge their skill level. Therefore, they are willing to pay accordingly. People need to feel that their work is valued, and employers, more or less, get what they pay for.

The most successful dental practices provide employees with additional incentives to promote continued practice growth and financial profitability. These incentives can be financial, in the form of bonuses or profit sharing plans, or they can consist of motivational strategies which provide the staff with a sense of pride and the desire to succeed.

Team members can be motivated by being provided with an opportunity to participate in decisions that relate to practice growth. It is important for staff members to have a sense of pride and ownership for their job, which encourages them to develop winning attitudes. Employees generally respond favourably when they feel that their opinions or suggestions have been listened to, considered, and respected. Dental team members can be valuable marketing tools. Creative endeavour and continued education should be encouraged and applauded. Thus, a continuing education program can be a staff incentive.

Dental office staff should reflect a positive and healthy image. Accordingly, instead of paying employees for "sick days," an incentive would be to pay them for being well, in other words, "wellness days." Employees who remain well all year could receive a bonus for their wellness days. This provides employees with positive reinforcement to encourage their continued good health. Of course, this should not penalize employees for unavoidable illness.

Employee benefit programs can be offered as an incentive, for example, an extended health care plan that includes prescriptions, vision care, and an employee dental plan. Because these benefit programs are costly to the dentist, they will likely have restrictive clauses and eligibility requirements.

Dental offices do not usually offer a pension plan. However, RRSPs (registered retirement savings plans) can be purchased under a group contract. This can provide the dentist with a tax shelter in the form of a deduction. The dentist and the employee can share in the contribution, enabling both parties to have the benefit of a tax deduction. The end result is a satisfied employee who has a sense of job security and a pension on retirement.

When the team is actively marketing and reinforcing the wellness theme, personal enthusiasm, job satisfaction, and ultimately job performance are increased. Working together to encourage group cohesiveness creates a pleasant atmosphere and opens the doors to creativity. This process makes staff feel that they are valued contributors to the practice and that their opinion is held in high regard. When the overall esteem of everyone in the office is enhanced, a positive office image prevails which makes each patient feel welcome. Enthusiasm is contagious. It is the art of feeling and easily expressing an intensity or excitement about dentistry that radiates an energetic feeling of interest to others.

ASSIGNMENT

1. Write a short essay describing how you would respond to the following conflicts:
   a. The hygienists have complained that they are often required to stay late because of improper appointment scheduling and they do not have time to prepare instruments between appointments.
   b. One of the dental assistants is upset because she discovered that someone else is making more money than she is.
2. Prepare a meeting agenda to discuss these issues.

CHAPTER TWENTY

WRITTEN COMMUNICATIONS

O B J E C T I V E

At the end of this chapter, the student will be able to identify and describe the following: standard letter styles, the correct use of punctuation and grammar, redundant wording, composition of a business letter, common spelling errors, and a strategy to improve grammar, spelling, and punctuation.

T O P I C S

- spelling improvement
- grammar
- parts of speech
- sentence structure
- punctuation
- letter styles

THE CHALLENGE OF COMMUNICATIONS

Written communications present a great challenge to the dental professional. The dental office administrator must represent the practice in a polished and professional manner at all times. Written communications do not allow the receiver the luxury of reading the body language of the sender to provide clarity to the message. Therefore, it is essential that written communications be clear, concise, complete, and correct. When an error appears in a written form of communication, subliminally this suggests that clinical errors may also be acceptable at that dental practice.

The purpose of developing a meaningful relationship between the dental office staff and the patient is to enhance the patient's level of trust. The level of trust increases when the staff are consistently professional and polished in each stage of treatment and follow-up.

Consistency in written communications also reassures the patient that he or she is dealing with highly educated and experienced dental health specialists.

The dental office administrator is expected to be a communications expert in addition to a dental health specialist. A basic understanding of English and a lot of common sense is all that is required to be an effective communicator. Clarity is achieved by using terms that are easily and quickly understood and that do not allow room for doubt or misinterpretation of the message.

Conciseness is saying what you have to say in the fewest possible words. The right letter or written communication can win back a disgruntled patient, reinforce the importance of follow-up dental care, enhance the public image of the office, eliminate unnecessary additional correspondence, and save time.

Methods of Spelling Improvement

One of the most obvious errors in written communications is spelling. Not everyone is a masterful speller, but there are some simple methods to follow to improve spelling proficiency. The following are some suggestions to develop good spelling habits:

- Study from lists of words you misspell. Keep a notebook of words that are difficult to spell and need to be looked up every time.
- Break down the words into the component parts, such as the prefix, root word, and suffix, as in dental terminology. Spell out the word letter by letter.
- Use mnemonic devices. A mnemonic device is a memory enhancer, such as basic spelling rules. For example, "*i* before *e* except after *c,* and when it sounds like *a* as in neighbour and weigh" or there are three *e*'s in therefore.
- Pronounce words correctly. Study the word to learn how its consonant and vowel sounds are spelled. Read the word aloud. Write the spelling of the word without looking at it. If a word is pronounced incorrectly, there is a greater risk of spelling it incorrectly. For example, "asprin" is how it is often pronounced, but *aspirin* is the correct spelling.

- Master spelling rules. There are many spelling rules that can be followed.
- Develop a habit of proofreading all documents very carefully. So elicit help from a friend to make certain that there are no errors. Many times an error is overlooked because it did not appear to be an error in the first place.

When in doubt, look it up.

Dictionary Usage

When a word has more than one spelling, the preferred spelling is usually listed first in the dictionary. The second spelling is known as the variant spelling. Use the preferred spelling first. Use the dictionary for the pronunciation of vowel sounds (i.e., the sound *aw* is usually represented by the circumflex ^, as in pôt). If there is anything unusual about the spellings of verbs ending with -*ed, -ing,* or -*s,* the spellings are stated at the beginning of verb definitions, as they are if the final consonant is doubled, as in *conferred* and *conferring.* If the emphasis is placed on the second syllable, as in *refer,* the consonant is doubled before adding the suffix.

A misspeller's dictionary can help if you look up a word by the way it sounds phonetically, and find the correct spelling; for example, the word sounds like *fasinate,* but is spelled *fascinate.*

Grammar

Occasionally the office administrator will need to correct grammatical errors, reword a phrase, or rearrange a sentence before sending out a document. All documentation that leaves the office should be letter perfect. Knowledge of correct grammar can be an extremely important asset, while the lack of it can be detrimental.

The following represents essential parts of speech:

Noun
Common or proper name of a person, place, thing, or idea. Example: **Susan** prefers **skirts** to **jeans.** *Susan* is the proper noun while *skirts* and *jeans* are common nouns.

Pronoun
Takes the place of a noun, for example, *he, she,* etc. A pronoun is a word used in place of a noun; it may be used in place of more than one noun.
Example: **You** and **she** run fast.

Personal Pronoun

Personal pronouns take the place of a noun. They can be used in one of three ways:

First person—the person talking about himself or herself.

Example: **I** took the book to **our** house.

Second person—the person being spoken to.

Example: **You** can keep **your** money.

Third person—the person being spoken about.

Example: **He** gave **his** letter to **them**.

Relative Pronoun

Relative pronouns are used to introduce nouns or noun clauses. They are also used in adjective clauses and use the words **who, whom, whose, which, that.**

Example: The book **that** I borrowed from the library was about the history of medicine.

Adjective

An adjective modifies a noun or pronoun. Example: That was an **unnerving** ride. They are **noisy.** Adjectives are used to make the meaning of the noun or pronoun more definitive.

Examples: **white** uniform

old method

weak muscles

Adjectives may also indicate which one:

Examples: **this** hospital

those books

that EKG

Or they may tell how many:

Examples: **five** doctors

two nurses

several aides

Verb

Shows action or state of being.

Examples: She **began** to **work.**

The nurse **is** happy.

The verb is a word that expresses action or otherwise helps to make a statement. There are two types of action verbs, but it is necessary only to identify them here as action verbs. Some action verbs, like **jump, sing,** and **shout,** can be seen or heard, but others cannot. Action verbs that cannot be seen or heard include **think, evaluate,** and **distrust.**

Examples: The doctor **injected** her. (This verb is seen.)

The patient **distrusts** him. (This verb is unseen.)

Linking verbs help to make a statement by serving as a link between two words. The most common of these are forms of the verb **be**.

Example: He **is** not the man he used **to be**.

Any verb phrase ending in **be** (**can be, will be**) or **been** (**had been, might have been**) is a form of the verb **be**. There are other common linking verbs such as **appear, become, feel, grow, remain, smell, sound, stay,** and **taste.**

Examples: The patient **feels** well.

The blood level **remains** constant.

The diagnosis **appears** to be correct.

Her condition **stays** the same.

The coffee **tastes** good.

Adverb

Modifies a verb, an adjective, or another verb.

Examples: Interns learn **quickly.**

Are doctors **always** right?

He jumps **quite** high.

An adverb is a word used to modify a verb, an adjective, or another adverb. It qualifies the meaning of words by answering the questions of **how, when, where,** or **to what extent.** Many adverbs end in **ly,** but certainly not all of them.

Example: She **always** arrives **too soon.**

An adverb may also modify other adverbs.

Example: The patient spoke **too quickly.** (**Quickly** is the adverb telling how the patient spoke. **Too** tells how quickly.)

Some adverbs modify adjectives.

Examples: Medicine companies have **fiercely** competitive prices. (modifies competitive)

Her patient was **exceptionally** brave. (modifies brave)

Preposition

Relates a noun or pronoun to another word.

Example: The balls are **in** the yard, **under** the tree, **near** the house.

Prepositions are words that combine with a noun or a pronoun to show a relationship to another word in the sentence.

Examples: The doctor rode **past** the hospital.

He parked **near** the hydrant and looked **across** the street.

At, after, by, for, from, in, of, on, since, to, and **until** are easily recognized prepositions.

There are many other commonly used prepositions:

about	besides	outside
above	between	over
across	beyond	past
against	concerning	through
along	down	toward
amid	during	under
among	except	underneath
around	inside	up
before	into	upon
behind	like	with
below	near	within

Conjunction

Joins words, phrases, or clauses.

Example: The doctor **and** nurse are a team.

The conjunction is probably the easiest part of speech to recognize. It joins words, phrases, or clauses that function in the same way or in a closely related way. There are three types of conjunctions: coordinating, correlating, and subordinating.

Coordinating conjunctions join equal parts of a sentence.

Example: She was tired, **yet** she stayed awake.

Many of the above words can be used as other parts of speech. You will recognize some that can be used as prepositions.

Sentence Structure

It is essential to understand correct sentence structure, grammar, and punctuation in order to compose business correspondence, prepare reports, or rearrange words without changing the meaning or tone of the communication. A sentence is a group of words, containing a **subject (noun or pronoun)** and a **predicate (verb)** that can stand alone as a complete thought.

The Subject

A sentence must refer to someone or something. This the **simple subject**.

Example: **Jane** assists the doctor. (simple subject)

A subject may be simple or complete. **Jane** is the simple subject; any added words that describe, identify, or explain more about Jane would be included in the **complete subject**.

Example: **Jane, the dental office administrator,** assists the doctor.
(complete subject)

The subject is the doer of the action.

The Predicate

A sentence must tell something about a person or thing. The word, or words, that do this are called the **predicate** and always contain a verb.

Example: Jane **assists.** (simple predicate)

The word **assists** tells us what Jane does. **Assists** is the simple predicate. Other words that describe the verb would be the complete predicate. They could tell how, when or where.

Example: Jane **bowls often at the City Bowl.** (complete predicate)

When speaking, we often tend to talk in incomplete sentences. These are called **fragmented sentences.** They are usually understood and accepted orally.

Examples: "Hi, Jane. Where have you been?"
"Doctor's office."
"What's wrong?"

In writing we must not do that. Since we cannot be seen or heard, the written words must convey the whole message. On paper we must express ourselves in complete sentences.

Example: The blanket covered.

Even with a subject and predicate, the above sentence is not a complete thought. There must be more.

Example: The blanket covered the patient.

This is a complete sentence.

Simple Sentences

Sentences may be structured in several ways. Some expressions are made in **simple sentences.** These are easy and basic to all others.

Example: The patient was referred for a cephalometric x-ray.

Compound Sentences

A **compound sentence** makes two separate statements that are closely related.

Example: The patient was sent for a cephalometric x-ray; she also had to have an orthodontic consultation.

Complex Sentences

A **complex sentence** can be long and involved. It can also be compound-complex, and can sometimes be divided into two or more sentences.

Example: The patient is going very early to have a chest x-ray; she is also ordered to get a CBC at the same time, and while she is there, she might as well make an appointment for an upper GI series.

This could easily be broken down into two or three sentences.

Punctuation

Punctuation is necessary in all written communication in order to make it understandable and clear. The reader must be able to identify when one thought ends and another begins. Voice inflection and intensity of expression or feeling can be changed or communicated by punctuation. Punctuation discussed here will include sentence endings, commas, colons, semicolons, and hyphens.

Each punctuation mark is used for clarity. How much punctuation is enough? One of the basic rules of thumb for punctuation is **when in doubt, leave it out**. Too much punctuation can distract the reader by creating too many pauses. Also, if you cannot justify why you are placing punctuation where you are, do not put it in. This does not mean that you should not punctuate your written communications properly; it simply means you should not ruin your communication with too much punctuation.

Period, Question Mark, or Exclamation

Every sentence or statement will have a mark of punctuation at the end. A sentence that **tells** something has a **period**.

Example: The doctor's diagnosis was unexpected.

A sentence that **asks a question** has a **question mark** at the end.

Example: Was your appointment today?

A sentence that instructs or commands will have a period. If the command or instruction is urgent, it can end with an **exclamation mark**.

Examples: Nurse, please close the door.
　　　　　Susan, close that door now!

A sentence that exclaims with enthusiasm or emotion also ends with an exclamation mark.

Commas

Commas can cause many problems unless you know a few simple rules. Too much punctuation is as confusing as too little. This is one of the most common errors that occur when one is learning proper punctuation. Commas create a slight pause when reading. If you are unsure of whether or not you have too many commas, read sentences aloud inserting a deliberate pause each time that you encounter a comma. If your communication lacks clarity because of too many commas, take them out. This is when common sense plays a major role in effective written communications.

Some basic rules for commas are as follows:

Dates require a comma between the day and the year.

Example: March 29, 1994

If the year is not followed by a semicolon, period, question mark, or exclamation mark to end the sentence, a comma is placed after the year also.

Examples: On March 29, 1993, Sharri was born. On July 30, 1993, she cut her first tooth. She took her first steps on December 15, 1994.

Commas and Places

Commas are placed after the following:

The name of a town, village, or city.

Examples: Calgary, Alberta
Toronto, Ontario
Regina, Saskatchewan

Post office box number or rural route number.

Example: R.R. 3, Box 5103, Beamsville, Ontario, L9K 9K9

Commas in a Series

Use commas to separate a group of **related** words in a series.

Example: Cynthia, Marian, and Alice have decided to become nurses. They have a lot of studies in biology, chemistry, anatomy, and physiology.

Commas are used to separate **related phrases** in a series.

Example: The hospital is an organization governed by a board of directors, the overseeing administrator, and a group of doctor trustees.

Commas are used to separate **subordinate clauses** in a series.

Example: The student doctors will pass their tests if they take good notes, if they study hard, and if they get a good night's sleep.

The last comma is left off if the last two items in a series are joined together.

Examples: The nurses' club elected a president, a vice-president, and a secretary-treasurer.
The patient's operation consisted of a face lift, a tummy tuck and liposuction.

Independent Clauses

An independent clause contains a noun and a verb and can stand alone, similar to a sentence. However, it is not a complete thought. Short independent clauses may be separated by commas, but semicolons usually separate them.

Example: As doctors interested in physical fitness, we jogged, we swam, and we went to the gym.

When an independent clause is joined with a conjunction, a comma should precede the conjunction. An easy way to remember this is by using the acronym FANBOYS. If two independent clauses are joined by FOR, AND, NOR, BUT, OR, YET, or SO, then use a comma.

Example: The patient needs to be referred to Dr. Smith for a consultation, and she will require a cephalometric x-ray for diagnostic purposes.

Nonessential Clauses and Phrases

A nonessential clause is one that is not essential to the sentence but adds extra information or explains something more. This also applies to an appositive, which restates the noun. These clauses are set off by commas and could be omitted without changing the meaning of the sentence.

Example: Mark Hatfield, now studying to be an intern, works with Dr. Stone.

Essential clauses, on the other hand, do not need commas. Most of these clauses are introduced by **that**.

Example: The student books that are required are known as texts.

Commas Separate Introductory Phrases

Commas are used after such words as **yes, no, well**, and **why** when they begin a sentence. Use a comma after an introductory phrase, series of phrases, or introductory adverb clause.

Examples: In the darkness, by the light of the moon, the situation appeared romantic.

As you can see by my last memo, I still await your reply.

After they took a three-and-a-half-hour exam, 12 of the students stayed up all night.

Semicolons

The semicolon says to pause just a little longer than you do for a comma, but less than is necessary for a period. There are four reasons to use a semicolon:

1. Between independent clauses if they are not joined by a conjunction. This is especially true if the clauses are very closely connected.

   Example: Ima Love was elected president of the Nurses' Association; she truly deserved the recognition.

2. Between independent clauses, when joined by any of these words: **for example, for instance, that is, accordingly, nevertheless, however, furthermore, consequently, therefore, hence.**

   Example: Only two people came for the CPR class; consequently, the class was cancelled.

3. To separate independent clauses joined by a coordinating conjunction, if there are commas in the clause.

   Example: The disease of chlamydia, left untreated in men, may cause sterility; but, in women, it can lead to PID.

4. Between items in a series that already contain commas.

   Example: There are famous hospitals in all of these cities: Hamilton, Ontario; Ottawa, Ontario; and Toronto, Ontario.

Colons

Whether the text says it or not, a colon means "notice what is following." It is used as below:

1. To note what follows.

   Example: The nursing students were allowed four pieces of equipment in their exam area: stethoscopes, blood pressure cuffs, thermometers, and wrist watches.

2. Before a long, formal statement or quotation.

   Example: Psychologists tell us: "The bad taste of cold coffee may be more in your head than in your mug."

3. In certain conventional situations. Between the hour and the minutes in writing time.

   Examples: 8:20 a.m.

              9:50 p.m.

   After the salutation of a **business** letter.

   Examples: Dear Dr. Stitchem:

              Gentlemen:

              To Whom It May Concern:

Quotation Marks

Quotation marks are most often used to show that someone's exact words are being used. Quotation marks are always in pairs, one at the beginning of the quote and one at the end.

Note: A direct quote will begin with a capital letter.

Examples: The nurse asked, "When do we get our uniforms?"

The doctor said jokingly, "A stitch in time saves nine"; however, it sounded strange coming from a surgeon.

Apostrophes

The apostrophe is used with a noun or a pronoun to indicate ownership or relationship. In English, you indicate the possessive case by adding "'s", or sometimes merely an apostrophe, to the noun. Plural words ending in s usually require only an apostrophe.

Examples: The nurse's uniform. (one nurse)

the nurses' schedule. (more than one nurse)

The most common use of apostrophes is in contractions where letters have been omitted.

Examples: I have—I've

you are—you're

it is—it's

is not—isn't

do not—don't

have not—haven't

The use of contractions, although common in everyday speech, is not generally accepted in written communications. Therefore, if the dentist dictates something like: "I've referred Mrs. Smith to the Fracture Clinic for further x-rays," you should type: "**I have** referred Mrs. Smith...." In other words, write contractions out in full.

Hyphens

Hyphens are used for two reasons. The first is to divide words at the end of a line and the second is to join the parts of compound words. Many word processing programs will provide the typist with a "word wrap" or "hyphenation" feature; however, if it is necessary to hyphenate words, some simple rules should be followed:

Always divide between syllables. If you don't know where to divide, consult the dictionary.

Examples: doc-tor, ortho-dontist

Already hyphenated words should be divided only at the hyphen.

Example: self-destructive

happy-go-lucky

The second reason hyphens are used is to join the parts of compound words; however, the tendency is to make two words instead of the one-word compound.

Examples: present-day policy

up-to-date techniques

Compound numbers are also joined with hyphens.

Examples: this thirty-three-year-old woman

three-and-one-half

Use a hyphen in words with the prefixes **all, ex,** and **self** and with the suffix **elect.**

Examples: self-contained

ex-secretary

President-elect

Finally, when a compound or two-word adjective precedes the noun it modifies, it is hyphenated.

Examples: middle-class neighbourhood

first-time swimmer

Parentheses

Material added to a sentence, but not considered of major importance, is enclosed in parentheses. Punctuation marks that belong to the parenthetical material are placed within the parentheses. They are placed outside the parentheses when they belong to the sentence as a whole.

Examples: The patient was given numerous tests (Were they all necessary?) before being told there was nothing wrong. The nurse tried on numerous uniforms (all expensive) before deciding on one.

Letter Styles

The main components of a business letter are the following:

- letterhead
- date
- inside address
- attention line
- salutation
- reference line
- body of letter
- complimentary closing
- enclosures
- copies notation
- signature block and originator's and typist's initials.

The **letterhead** will include the name and address of the dental practice as well as the logo (if one exists) and possibly the telephone number of the office. The usual size of a letterhead is 2.5 cm.

The **date** is typed approximately two to four lines below the letter-head.

The **inside address** will appear approximately four lines below the date. It will include the name, address, city, and postal code of the recipient of the letter.

The **attention line** will appear approximately two lines below the inside address. You will capitalize the word "ATTENTION:" or you may use the abbreviation "ATT:"; in either case, you will follow this with a full colon. An attention line is used when the letter is going to an organization and being directed to a specific person. For example, if the letter is addressed to Canadian Dental Associates, but the letter is to be directed to Dr. Smith, then Dr. Smith's name will appear in the attention line.

The **salutation** appears approximately two lines below the attention line. The salutation is the greeting and usually begins with Dear. The salutation line may also begin with Gentlemen, Ladies, etc.

The **reference line** will appear approximately two lines below the salutation. This line is also called the subject line. In dental office communication this line usually contains the name of the patient to whom reference is being made. This line will begin with "RE:" typed in capitals and followed with a full colon, for example, "RE: Your patient Susan Smith." This line is helpful to the reader as it allows the recipient the opportunity to pull the patient's chart.

The **body** of the letter is usually single spaced. It appears approximately two lines below the reference line. The body of the letter usually contains approximately two paragraphs. A paragraph should consist of more than one sentence.

The **complimentary closing** appears approximately two lines below the last line in the body of the letter. The first word only of the complimentary closing is capitalized, for example, "Yours truly," "Sincerely," "Yours in the interest of dental health,".

The **signature block** will appear approximately four lines below the complimentary closing. This allows room for the signature. If the dentist is dictating the letter, then that is the name that will appear in the signature block. It is the dentist's preference as to whether the name should be preceded with Dr., or if it should be succeeded with the degrees held.

For example,

Dr. I. Jones, D.D.S.
Dr. J. Smith, B.Sc., D.D.S.
R. Gold, D.D.S.

A general guideline to follow is to list the degrees in the order that they have been obtained.

An **enclosure** line appears approximately two lines below the signature block and is used only if something is being enclosed. You can type the word "enclosure" or "encl." or indicate the number of pages enclosed or identify what is enclosed. The most commonly used notation is "encl."

The **complimentary copy** line will appear approximately two lines below the enclosure line if one exists; otherwise, it will be two lines below the signature block. This line will identify if copies have been forwarded to other parties. This line is identified with "cc:" followed by the names of people the copies will be sent to.

There are several styles of letters which can be used in written communication. The most commonly used letter style is full block style. This style is popular because of the efficiency and speed of word processing equipment.

The *full block style* is the easiest to remember as all lines begin at the left margin.

Modified block style is similar to block in that all lines begin at the left margin with the exception of the date, the complimentary closing, and the signature block; all of these begin at the middle. This letter style can also be modified to include beginning these lines at the right margin, or flush right. Modified block can be varied to include paragraph indentation.

The modified block format represents a slightly more time-consuming method of writing. The preferred letter style is full block with mixed punctuation.

Mixed punctuation indicates that there is punctuation present after the salutation and after the complimentary closing. The punctuation following a salutation should always be a full colon in business letters. A comma may be used in a personal letter. Mixed punctuation is the preferred style used in today's business letters.

Closed punctuation indicates that there is punctuation after every short line. Commas or periods are placed after the name, title, street address, etc. This punctuation style is more time-consuming and cumbersome; therefore, it is not preferred. If your dentist does prefer this method, it is recommended that you use modified block letter format.

Open punctuation indicates that there is no punctuation after any of the short lines, including the salutation and complimentary closing. Although this punctuation style certainly requires less time, it is not

EXHIBIT 20.1 **FULL BLOCK LETTER STYLE**

Dr. D. Kay
123 Bicuspid Street
Your City, Your Province
Postal Code

Date

Name of Recipient
Street Address
City, Province
Postal Code

ATTENTION: *(If the letter is addressed to an organization)*

Dear _____ :

RE:
(body of letter) _____
_____
_____
_____
_____
_____

Yours truly,

Dr. D. Kay, D.D.S.
Encl. *(only if something is enclosed)*
MM/sb *(initials of the person who dictated the letter and the person who typed the letter)*

preferred because of the aesthetic appearance of the letter—it looks as if something is missing.

It is acceptable to use any letter style with any style of punctuation. The preferred letter style, as previously mentioned, is full block style with mixed punctuation. Always remember to use a good quality bond paper and proofread the letter before submitting it for signature. If you are using a word processor that has a spell checker, be sure to spell check your document immediately upon completion.

EXHIBIT 20.2 MODIFIED BLOCK LETTER STYLE

Dr. D. Kay
123 Bicuspid Street
Your City, Your Province
Postal Code

Date

Name of Recipient
Street Address
City, Province
Postal Code

ATTENTION: *(If the letter is addressed to an organization)*

Dear _____:

RE:
(body of letter) ———————————————————————
————————————————————————————————
————————————————————————————————
————————————————————————————————
————————————————————————————————
————————————————————————————————
————————————————————————————

Yours truly,

Dr. D. Kay, D.D.S.

MM/sb

The spell check feature is convenient to use. However, if you have a software program that is from the United States, be aware of the differences in the spelling of certain words. In addition, do not be too reliant on the spell check feature as it will not check for correct context or grammar. Even if you do have a word processor that has a grammar check, it is still important to understand grammar basics in order to use it correctly. The same rule applies with the spell check feature; it is still important to know how to spell.

ASSIGNMENT

SENTENCE STRUCTURE

1. Read the sentences below and identify the simple subject and the simple predicate.

   a. The discovery of radium has been credited to Marie and Pierre Curie.

   b. As a student, Marie first discovered the rays of uranium.

   c. Marie was born in Poland in 1867.

   d. Pierre Curie, a Frenchman, was born in 1859.

2. Return to the activity you just finished. Now, draw one line under the complete subject. Draw two lines under the complete predicate.

PUNCTUATION

3. Rewrite the following sentences, placing commas where needed.

   a. Sharon Susan and Anthony plan to go to New York for a vacation.

   b. They plan among other things to study nutrition and health.

4. Rewrite the following sentences, putting in colons and semicolons where needed.

   a. Many people won't use bread however, it is a good source of protein, riboflavin, iron, and thiamine.

   b. Esther won the Miss Health Contest she certainly looked both healthy and beautiful.

5. Rewrite the following sentences using quotation marks where needed.

   a. Being in a hurry, the doctor said, Give me a ham on rye, and make it quick.

   b. Another customer asked, When do you have to return?

LETTER WRITING

6. Please type the following letter in full block style with mixed punctuation.

   To: Mrs. Marsha Mason, 123 Lane Way, Toronto, Ontario, L8K 4G1

   I would like to take this opportunity to thank you for your confidence in referring your friend, Mrs. Sally Strange, and her children, John and Debbie, to my office for treatment. My staff and I will make every attempt to justify the confidence you have shown in us during the treatment of Mrs. Strange and her family. Thank you again for your expression of confidence. Sincerely, Dr. M. Molar, B.Sc., D.D.S.

7. Please type the following letter in modified block style with open punctuation.

To: The Calgary Post, 123 Centre Street, Calgary, Alberta, K1A 5T7

I wish to apply for the position of Dental Office Administrator as advertised in yesterday's Calgary Post. I am enclosing my résumé outlining my educational qualifications and work experience to enable you to evaluate my credentials in relation to your specific job requirements. Should you wish additional information, or if you wish to arrange an interview with me, I am available at your convenience and can be reached at (403) 555–5214. Your assistance and consideration of my request is most appreciated.

CHAPTER TWENTY-ONE

ORGANIZATIONAL TECHNIQUES

OBJECTIVE

At the end of this chapter, the student will be able to identify and describe the following: an office procedures and protocol manual, methods of time organization, a monthly diary, and the importance of organizational goals.

TOPICS

- office procedures and protocol manual
- effective time management
- daily diary, chronological filing system
- goal setting

PROCEDURES AND PROTOCOL MANUAL

Many dental practices may perform similar functions; however, the administrative duties differ in each office. A procedures and protocol manual describes in detail how each job is performed and what the expected outcome is. The process of developing a procedures manual may initially appear to be time-consuming, but in many cases it can be a mechanism to identify redundancy or overlapping of tasks.

A procedures manual is a reference book which should be easily accessible. A job description for each position can be helpful in the event that an employee is absent. Substitute staff can then identify and prioritize duties that are to be undertaken and follow the instructions contained in the manual.

Development of this manual can assist employees in cultivating and maintaining excellent organizational skills by identifying the duties they are responsible for and prioritizing them. This information can be a valuable tool for salary negotiations. Astute business people are focusing on efficiency and cost effectiveness by restructuring the job responsibilities of employees. A dental office administrator should take a personal interest in reducing wasted time and money. The procedures and protocol manual should be updated regularly, at least once a year, to incorporate any changes that have been made (e.g., changes in legislation) and to keep the information current.

A procedures and protocol manual can be helpful when hiring new staff members. It will clearly define the job responsibilities for each position, thereby assisting the interviewer in determining which skills match the job and salary range. This definition is also helpful when designing a newspaper advertisement for the job opening. The manual can be helpful for training purposes or orientation, and will assist a new employee to prioritize tasks so as not to become overwhelmed.

Some topics to include in your procedures and protocol manual are the following:

- detailed emergency procedures
- insurance form completion
- predeterminations
- Electronic Data Interchange transactions
- infection control
- transfer of records
- informed consent
- banking
- recall system

One of the most important functions of a procedures and protocol manual is to identify where emergency equipment is located within the office. All staff should be familiar with the location of emergency equipment and also how to use it. Periodically, the expiry dates, inspection dates, and condition of all emergency equipment should be checked. The dental office administrator should chronologically file a reminder card to check emergency equipment.

When emergencies occur in a dental office, every staff member should know what to do. Most people will remain calm if they have a specific job to do. Panic in the office will create chaos, which could have a devastating effect. All staff members should be trained in first aid and cardiopulmonary resuscitation.

EXHIBIT 21.1 **TASK PRIORITY LIST**

PRIORITIES	
0745	take messages and attend morning staff meeting
0800	open office
0815	check for postdated cheques, produce recall list and follow-up calls
0830	prepare list of confirmation calls
0900	begin confirmation calls for next day
1130	pull charts for next day, check for premeds
1330	photocopy schedules and colour code for next day
1430	prepare bank deposit
1500	call patients who need recare appointments
1530	file charts
1600	balance daysheet

Master Copies of Forms

Master copies of each of the office forms that are used for transferring records, consent for treatment, and financial arrangements can be kept in the procedures manual for easy reference. These forms can be photocopied easily if needed.

CHRONOLOGICAL FILING SYSTEM

A chronological filing system is one of the dental office administrator's most valuable tools. It can be set up using 12.7 cm by 7.6 cm (3" × 5") cards and dividers with tabs that are labelled 1 to 31 in a small file box. Each divider represents a day of the month. Each day upon arrival at the office, simply pull out the card for that particular day. Among other things, this is an excellent storage place for postdated cheques, which have been stamped with the restrictive endorsement stamp.

File notations can include follow-up on patients who are in active treatment, predeterminations, and delinquent accounts. A card can be inserted on the dates that automatic debits will be taken out of the bank account. On or before the 15th of each month, you should file a reminder to submit the payroll deductions for the previous month. If the 15th falls on a weekend, then the card should be moved to a few days before. You may also appreciate a card telling you when the payroll needs to be done.

The chronological file (also known as a 1 to 31 file) is such a helpful tool that you may decide to incorporate the procedures and protocol manual into it. You can type each procedure on a card and file it behind the day the procedure should be done. Once again, this would be an excellent tool for training new employees.

Separate cards would be useful for telephone procedures or scripts, procedures for ordering premedication from a pharmacy, and emergency procedures including where emergency equipment is located and when it was last inspected.

Recall Cards

Recall cards to be mailed to patients should be filed in a chronological filing system such as the 1 to 31 file. Refer to Chapter 10 to review the advance recall system.

FOLLOW-UP BINDER

Predeterminations or estimates are typically prepared when the dentist recommends treatment to a patient. At that time, the patient understands the necessity for the treatment and is prepared to make a commitment to complete it. It is mandatory that the dental office

EXHIBIT 21.2 **SAMPLE CARD FOR CHRONOLOGICAL FILE**

15

Receiver General Remittance

Go to bank before 3:00 p.m.

Call Mrs. Smith, follow-up with perio

administrator follow up with the patient in a timely manner. If too much time is allowed to pass, the patient may feel that the treatment is not important or perhaps not necessary.

A copy of the predetermination should be retained in a three-ring binder at the front counter. This will allow the administrator to make follow-up calls during the quiet times at the office. Never file the copy in the patient's chart as it may be overlooked there and lost income for the dentist will result.

File the copies of the predeterminations in a chronological order and allow approximately four to five weeks for approval. From time to time, patients may neglect to submit the predetermination to their insurance company and will appreciate a reminder.

The follow-up binder can be used to remind you to follow up on a variety of things, including delinquent accounts.

INSURANCE CODE REFERENCE SHEET

Every office should have a reference sheet listing treatment codes that are commonly used along with prices. The administrator will save time if codes do not have to be looked up in the fee guide. This reference should be located out of the patients' view but easily accessible to staff.

SETTING GOALS

A successful dental office administrator will enjoy his or her career more in a well-organized environment. Careful planning of the day-to-day operations will help to minimize the stress level within the dental office. Clearly defined duties and responsibilities will help to put everything into perspective and into order of priority. Preparing a daily objective or goal is a way to facilitate this process. It is important, however, to remain flexible enough to be prepared for unexpected changes or emergencies. Setting daily goals is the first step to creating a strategy for achievement. Setting many short term goals will place you on the path toward your long term goals.

ASSIGNMENT

1. Prepare a 1 to 31 chronological file using 12.7 cm × 7.6 cm (3″ × 5″) cards including reminders and dates.

CHAPTER TWENTY-TWO

THE JOB SEARCH

OBJECTIVE

At the end of this chapter, the student will be able to identify and describe the following: a professional résumé and cover letter, strategy for the job search, interviewing techniques, fears that employers face when hiring a new employee, and how to respond to those fears.

TOPICS

- skills, attendance, and punctuality
- attitude
- expectations
- rejection
- skills analysis/inventory
- your résumé and its purpose
- the cover letter
- the interview, interview questions
- employee fears
- salary negotiations

WHAT EMPLOYERS EXPECT

The first step toward a successful job search is to understand what is expected of the employment candidate. In other words, what are employers looking for? Dentistry is a service industry which is highly competitive and demanding. Rapid technological changes as well as changes to the Canadian economy have created an environment in which education beyond the high school level is essential. What this means to the job candidate is that employers are looking for employees well trained in their area of expertise who will make a strong contribution to the practice.

Skills

It important to be prepared for the competition when campaigning for a position. There are usually many people applying for few jobs. Employers will, therefore, recruit very carefully. They will begin by looking for solid basic skills in personal presentation, reading, writing, spelling, and mathematics. Shortcomings in these areas are obvious in the workplace, yet the recruitment process may not always identify the weakness.

Candidates who have a more diversified skill base have a greater chance for success. Many dental professionals will look for an employee who is flexible and has skills that are transferable, for example, one with both clinical and business skills. They will look for an employee who is willing to learn new things and adapts easily to change. In today's unpredictable employment market, it is important to have an attitude that change is positive.

Employers will look for an employee who has the ability to concentrate and take direction. A short attention span is a very unfortunate attribute. Every job contains some degree of detailed repetition and it becomes a challenge to remain focused.

Attendance and Punctuality

Attendance and punctuality are areas of great concern to employers. They need employees who are reliable. Employers will enquire about the attendance record of the candidate with previous employers. A good attendance record indicates that the applicant is reliable, enthusiastic, and willing to learn.

Punctuality and consistent attendance demand a degree of self-discipline. If a great deal of time was missed in the past due to illness, perhaps the applicant is not physically able to handle the job. A poor record may also indicate that the applicant does not reflect the healthy attitude that is required in a dental practice. Some illnesses are impossible to avoid; however, a healthy lifestyle can help to prevent many serious illnesses. If an employee misses work, it affects every member of the dental team. If this behaviour is repeated, team members, as well as the dentist, may become resentful and irritated.

Never be late for an interview; it creates a poor first impression. Common courtesy is highly visible behaviour. In the dental profession, punctuality is not just a courtesy, it is mandatory. The dentist's schedule is critically important to the practice. Being late displays disrespect for the dentist's time.

ATTITUDE

Have realistic expectations when you begin your job search. Do not expect to be Chief Executive Officer in the first three months. Be willing to demonstrate initiative and think through problems and to proceed accordingly. Do not expect employers to spend a lot of time training, coaching, and encouraging.

A mature attitude is necessary, one that is based on self-discipline and emotional control. Employers are looking for cooperative and strong contributors who are basically happy people. Personal happiness is one of the main ingredients to career success. A successful dental office administrator will recognize the importance of a well-balanced personal, physical, emotional, and professional life.

A SYSTEMATIC APPROACH TO THE JOB SEARCH

No one owes you a job; you have to fight for it using every skill at your disposal. You will be facing competition. It is important to be prepared and to make your résumé and cover letter stand out from the crowd. You must "sell" yourself to the potential employer. This is your opportunity to put your best foot forward and learn what works and what does not.

Successful organizations hire winners. If you are confident with your skills and abilities, it will be apparent to the person responsible for hiring. If you are feeling insecure and unsure of your abilities, then why should the employer feel any differently about you? A confident and happy person is attractive to the potential employer. A positive attitude reassures the employer and creates a sense of trust. If you do not feel confident, act as if you do. Everyone has butterflies; you must teach yours to fly in formation!

Rejection

The greater the number of avenues for employment that you explore, the better your chances for success. Expect it to take time. Expect rejection. You have no control over some of the reasons why you may not be hired for the job. It may be for a reason that you will never know. It could be simply because of an employer's screening method for a great number of applicants. It could also be that you are competing with someone who has more experience or training. All that you can do is present yourself in the best possible light, be honest and confident about your ability, and keep trying. Do not let rejection devastate you or impede your progress.

Make a full-time job out of trying to find a job. Do not just depend on one or two sources for employment leads. Explore a variety of avenues and do not be afraid to apply to dental offices or companies that interest you, even if they are not advertising. Not all job opportunities are advertised; in fact, many jobs can be obtained through personal referrals or through friends. If you are due for a dental appointment, talk to your dentist and describe the interesting course that you have just completed. Ask your dentist about job opportunities as a dental office administrator; this shows interest and enthusiasm. You must assume the management of your own job search. Get motivated!

Planning the Strategy

Avenues to Explore

- Newspaper advertisements—do not depend on advertisements alone, as many job openings are not advertised.
- Professional placement services—Remember that a placement service cannot legally charge the applicant a fee. If you are told that there is a fee, *do not use that service.*
- Word-of-mouth—talk to your friends, family, dentist, etc. Let them know what type of job you are looking for.
- Cold calls—Map out an area that is close to home, reasonable driving distance, or on a public transit route and drop off your résumé and cover letter to dental offices in your area. Remember to be dressed professionally at all times and to smile! If possible, ask if you can have the dentist's business card to follow up.
- Canada Employment Centre—Check the local office on a regular basis.
- Local library—Do some research on a company (perhaps a company that deals with dental insurance) that you are interested in and submit an application. A cover letter that focuses on specific

aspects of the company will attract the attention of the employer and show a lot of initiative.

The important thing to remember is to set a goal and define a strategy to achieve the goal. In other words, plan your job search schedule and map out your objectives. A typical day, for example, may include dropping off résumés and cover letters early in the morning. When you return home, make follow-up phone calls regarding résumés that were delivered the previous day. Look in the local newspaper and prepare more résumés and cover letters. Later in the afternoon, prepare and send thank-you notes to the offices that have granted you an interview and make follow-up phone calls. This helps the dentist to remember you and it displays courtesy. It is also an excellent reminder to let the dentist know that you are still seeking employment. Keep in mind that it is a "numbers" game. The more avenues that are explored and the more résumés that are submitted, the more chances you will have.

Who Are You? A Skills Analysis

The process of looking for employment is an opportunity for you to identify your strengths and weaknesses, take stock, reflect on past achievements, and bolster your confidence. Every time you go into a job interview, you must be able to tell an employer convincingly what you have to offer. You must know your skills and abilities and be able to present them in a clear and concise format. Preparing a skills inventory assists you to identify your own personal strengths and weaknesses.

Identify what your greatest strength is or what do you most enjoy doing, such as human relations, decision making, taking instruction, attending to the needs of people, exchanging information, coaching, instructing, organizing, or planning. Then identify your second greatest strength, and continue to rank the things that you most enjoy doing and that you are good at.

A good employer knows that unless an employee has enthusiasm for his or her work, the quality of that work will always suffer. People rarely enjoy something that they do badly. A bad employer will not care whether you enjoy a particular task, only whether you know how to do it. If your time is spent pursuing what gives you the greatest joy, you will be certain to do it well. This will result in quality job performance and overall job satisfaction.

Constructing a professional résumé is an opportunity to perform a skills analysis. This process will help to organize the information for your résumé, prepare for interviews, set goals, identify your strengths, and prepare to realize your potential. It will help you to identify your long term goals and create strategy or a mental map toward them.

THE RÉSUMÉ

A résumé should contain a *brief* account of your employment and educational history along with any additional qualifications. An effective résumé and cover letter can open the door to opportunity and lead you to an interview. Employers will often screen résumés to eliminate those that are ineffective or contain errors of *any* kind (i.e., typographical or spelling errors). Your résumé provides you with the opportunity to present yourself in the best possible light. If the best that you can do includes spelling or typing errors, then the employer may eliminate you from the selection process.

All of the information that the employer can learn about you before meeting you is contained in your résumé. A potential employer will typically spend three to five minutes "skimming" your résumé before deciding whether to further explore your potential.

The résumé should be professional in appearance and typed on a good quality bond paper. Office supply stores usually carry such paper. Avoid using paper that is too brightly coloured or flowery in appearance. Although your résumé will stand out, unusual paper may create a negative impression so that you will not be taken seriously.

Functions of the Résumé

One of the primary purposes of the résumé is to get you invited for an interview. Once invited, it will help to set the agenda for the meeting. This allows the interviewer to have a starting point for specific questions. An agenda will also help the interviewer to stay on track.

Once the interview has been completed, the résumé is a tangible reminder of it. Many interviewers jot down notes during the interview. You should try not to let that be a distraction. It usually indicates that the employer is interested and it helps jog the interviewer's memory when you have left.

Basic Points for the Résumé
1. Keep it brief. Do not write a story. If employers have to "dig" for information, they may choose not to.

2. There are many ways to put a résumé together, all correct, but there is no perfect way to complete a résumé. It is a representation of you as an individual and should reflect your distinctive qualities.

3. Point form is preferred as it is less time-consuming. Point form helps employers get to the necessary information quickly.

4. Reverse chronological order is preferred. List your work and educational history from the most current to the least. Do not go too far back in your history (public school, for example).

5. Include dates with your work and educational history. It is important for the employer to identify how relevant your work history or education is to the current job that is being advertised. For example, a part-time course in microcomputer applications that was taken 10 years ago would not provide the appropriate skill base for the current job market.

6. Include a telephone number where you can be reached. If you do not have an answering machine or cannot be reached during the day, an alternative phone number would help you not to miss those important calls. You may wish to ask a close friend or relative to help with this.

7. Do not just send out one résumé and wait for a reply. Send out many along with the appropriate cover letters. Make sure that they reflect your professional attitude and help the employer to take you seriously.

8. Include a covering letter.

9. Include references. Although opinions may vary regarding this point, it is preferable to have at least one or two references listed on the résumé that include telephone numbers. Interviewers may call the people listed to obtain an evaluation of past performance or perhaps a character reference. If you have a written reference, attach a copy to the résumé.

The Cover Letter

The cover letter should be clear, concise, and correct. In order for the letter to draw the attention of the reader, it should be "you" oriented. Such a letter makes a positive impression and suggests a sense of cooperation. This will attract the reader's attention and promote a positive response.

The letter should invite the reader to examine the résumé and schedule an interview. It should contain a positive tone and wording, suggesting that the message is relevant and requires a response.

EXHIBIT 22.1 SAMPLE COVER LETTER

To Whom It May Concern:

I wish to explore the possibility of obtaining a position as Dental Office Administrator within your practice. I will be relocating to your area in the near future and would like to offer your business office a strong contribution and personal commitment.

As you can see by my attached résumé, I am well qualified for this position and would appreciate the opportunity to discuss this with you.

Should you feel that your practice would benefit from an experienced employee who is dedicated and enthusiastic, please feel free to contact me at (905) 555-2211. I will be happy to meet with you for an interview at your convenience.

Thank you for your consideration and I look forward to hearing from you.

Sincerely,

Your name
Dental Office Administrator

THE INTERVIEW

The job interview can be stressful for the candidate being interviewed, but it is equally tension producing for the employer. The interviewer has a very limited amount of time to determine if the applicant will be the right person for the job and will fit well into the practice. In order to prepare for the interview, the applicant should begin by preparing questions to ask the interviewer.

For example,

- What does this job involve?
- Do my skills match this job?

In addition, there are questions to ask yourself during and after the interview.

- Is the atmosphere friendly and welcoming to new staff members?
- If it is a good match, how can I persuade the employer to hire me?

EXHIBIT 22.2 **SAMPLE RÉSUMÉ**

Susan Jones
101 Main Street
Toronto, Ontario
L9N 1P8
Telephone : (905) 555-1211
Alternate: (905) 555-2121

CAREER OBJECTIVE:
To obtain a position as Dental Office Administrator in a progressive practice where I can utilize my skills and potential and offer a strong contribution.

EMPLOYMENT HISTORY:

July 1986–current	DR. M. MOLAR, 44 Bicuspid Lane
	Toronto, Ontario
	L4N 1Z3
Position:	Dental Office Administrator
	• Effective appointment scheduling
	• Ensuring patient comfort and optimal care
	• Patient flow
	• Collection procedures
	• Computer data entry
	• Completion of insurance forms

EDUCATION:

Current	Dental Administration College of Canada, 2 Education Lane, Toronto, Ontario, M7K 3L9
	Diploma—Dental Office Administrator
1980	Grade 12 Diploma
	Central School, Toronto, Ontario

REFERENCES: Mrs. Judy Jones,
                         Instructor, Dental Administration College of Canada
                         (905) 555-7789

                         Additional references available upon request

It is essential to present yourself professionally. Although you may consider this to be common sense it is not always common practice. Put yourself in the position of the employer who is going to hire you. What would you be looking for?

Be on time for the interview. In fact, arrive a little early, but not too early. If you are late, forget it. Even though there may be subsequent interviews, this is your one and only chance to make a good first impression.

Bring an extra copy of your résumé with you. The interviewer will have a copy; however, it may be temporarily misplaced or unavailable at the time of the interview. This displays good organizational skills on your part.

Demonstrate your most valuable skill—communication. Practise and perfect your verbal and nonverbal communication skills. Use proper grammar and speak clearly. Avoid slang terms and never use profanity.

Eye contact is essential as it displays sincerity and honesty. The interviewer will be watching for subtle clues that will help him or her decide if you should be hired. Keep your gestures open and show interest in the practice and enthusiasm about the dental profession. Do not giggle or chew gum.

Most interviewers understand that you will be nervous and will expect you to be; that is normal. Taking a few deep breaths, breathing in very slowly and out very slowly, will help to increase the level of oxygen to the brain. This creates a very calming and soothing effect on the body. Try to be discreet when performing this deep breathing exercise.

Plan and prepare what you are going to wear the day before the interview. Make sure that your clothing is clean and professional in appearance. Select clothing that suits you and that indicates to the interviewer that you are to be taken seriously. Clothing that is too casual or provocative is not appropriate for a professional job interview.

CONCERNS OF THE POTENTIAL EMPLOYER

Employers or interviewers are also nervous during an interview. They have many concerns and fears when selecting the appropriate employee for their office. An interviewer has a limited amount of time to discover as much information as possible about you and must try to find out if your background or attitude would make you a bad choice.

For your interview to be successful, it is recommended that you address the employer's concerns as much as possible and as soon as you have an opportunity. In fact, if you can pre-empt the questions, you will reassure the interviewer that you are the appropriate choice for the position.

For example, an employer may want to know about your attendance at your last job or during the course that you completed. Address the concern before the employer tries to extract the information. Although an employer cannot exclude you from the selection process based on whether or not you have small children, this factor may be an underlying concern. The employer may be afraid that you will miss too much work if a child becomes ill. If you do have small children, address the employer's fear by explaining that you have excellent daycare arranged and an emergency plan in place in the event that your child becomes ill.

The following is a list of other concerns that employers consider when hiring and suggestions of how to address them:

1. If you are hired, you will not be able to do the job. Do your skills and experience match the position? *Emphasize your skills that match the position that was advertised.*

2. If hired, you won't put in a full working day and you will frequently be off sick. Employers question attendance and punctuality because they need dependable employees in good health. *Stress your perfect attendance and how you pride yourself on punctuality.*

3. If hired, you will only stay a few months until something better comes along. If there are many job changes on your résumé or your long term goals are to do something other than dental office administration, you could be using this position as a stepping stone along your career path. The employer may also be concerned that as soon as something does not go your way, you will leave the position. *Emphasize your willingness to offer a strong contribution and commitment to the practice.*

4. It will take you too long to master the job. Employers do not have the time or resources to spend on lengthy training periods. They need an employee who is eager to learn and can catch on quickly. *Display your enthusiasm for dentistry and your desire to learn. Emphasize how quickly you have mastered a particular skill (perhaps a computer program).*

5. You will not get along with others and will cause personality conflicts, which can be devastating to a well-organized team environment. One "bad apple" can disrupt the entire office. *Emphasize how much you enjoy working with others and demonstrate your ability to work as part of a team.*

6. You will do only the minimum required. Some employees judge the amount of effort they are willing to extend by the amount of their paycheque. Employers are looking for people who are willing to give of themselves and display initiative. *Let the employer know that you understand that emergencies happen in dental offices and you don't mind staying late when necessary and coming in early to prepare for the day.*

7. You will always have to be told what to do next. An employee who requires constant supervision can cost the practice valuable time and resources. It is more cost effective to hire an employee who is a self-starter and is able to work with minimal supervision. *Emphasize that you work well alone or with a team and that you are honest and dependable.*

8. You have a disruptive character flaw—you spread dissension throughout the office, display a poor attitude, create negativity, gossip, or are dishonest or incompetent. A person with any of these negative characteristics can be a burden on any practice. Staff members will tend to avoid that person and so will patients. *Display a calm and mature attitude and speak positively of others, particularly past employers.*

Employers care about your past. However, they are more concerned about your future. Be natural and polite, and dress well (conservatively). Make it clear that you are healthy and maintain good posture and a positive, confident attitude. Smile and show genuine interest in the job being offered. At the end of the interview, thank the employer for taking the time to see you and conclude with a handshake. You may or may not be offered the position, and the employer may have other applicants to interview.

Every interview, whether it is good or bad, should be looked at as a learning experience. Look for the positive aspect of each interview and analyze what you feel worked and what did not. We learn best by our mistakes, so take the time to determine where changes could be made. This will help you to prepare for the next interview.

SALARY NEGOTIATIONS

Prepare yourself for the negotiation process by knowing what you expect your salary to be before you go for the interview and be willing to *negotiate*. Always think carefully before accepting a job. Even if the salary is lower than expected, the job may be an opportunity for you to prove your ability and worth at that office and gain experience. Consider all aspects of the job, including the location of the office, the hours, job responsibilities, and benefits, in addition to salary. Then feel free to ask the interviewer how your work will be evaluated and when. Once the interviewer has had an opportunity to see how quickly you learn and you have proved your overall value to the practice, you will be in a good position to negotiate a salary increase.

Salary is usually an issue that is addressed by the interviewer. It is a very important aspect of the interviewing process; however, it is not recommended that the dental office administrator address the issue too early in the interview. Allow the interviewer time to bring up salary. Some dental offices have a definite salary structure and benefits program and some do not.

If you are asked what your salary expectations are, state clearly and confidently what you expect and let the interviewer know that you are willing to negotiate. It is helpful to do some investigating to see if pay scales differ according to geographical location or job responsibilities. It is not advisable to request anything less than the average rate. Remember to maintain a standard of professionalism and not to attempt to undercut other applicants. This is considered an unethical practice that will ultimately reflect badly on the professional dental office administrator.

Follow-Up

Send a follow-up note to thank the interviewer for seeing you even if you are not hired. A thank-you note should be sent two or three days after the interview. Briefly, the note should thank the interviewer for allowing you the opportunity to discuss the position and restate your interest in the job. A follow-up note is a very effective way of reminding the interviewer of who you are and it will make your interview stand out.

Once You Are Hired

It is important for a successful dental office administrator to maintain a high standard of skill and integrity as well as to continue professional growth. Continued education is an important aspect of personal and professional development. It is helpful for the dental office administrator to become involved with local professional associations within the dental community. These associations provide dental professionals with information about continued education, seminars, symposia, and so on. They also provide a valuable opportunity for networking, learning from others who have similar experiences and ideas to share.

Finally, continue to set goals which will lead you on a triumphant journey toward a happy and prosperous career.

ASSIGNMENT

1. Prepare a skills inventory. Identify the skills that you most enjoy.
2. Prepare a résumé and cover letter.
3. Create a job search plan. Consider where you would most like to work.

CHAPTER TWENTY-THREE

COMPUTERS IN DENTAL OFFICES

OBJECTIVE

At the end of this chapter, the student will be able to identify and describe the following: the role of computerization in the dental office, hardware and software, and operating systems. The student will also be able to develop computer literacy and describe how a computer can assist with daily operations in a dental office as a valuable organizational tool.

TOPICS

- definition of a computer
- fear of learning computer skills
- needs analysis
- hardware/software
- operating systems
- daily activities
- care and maintenance

COMPUTER LITERACY

Technology has become such an integral part of our daily living that computer literacy is no longer a luxury, it is essential knowledge. A reasonable understanding of computer applications is now necessary to make a telephone call, set a digital clock, perform personal banking procedures, or even to solve the mystery of the VCR. The advance that have been made in computer technology in recent years can be overwhelming. Fortunately, computers and computer programs have become increasingly user friendly and provide considerable interaction with the operator.

Although traditionally there has been reluctance to convert to using computers as functional business tools, many successful businesses now realize the benefits of storing and manipulating large amounts of data with great efficiency. The steadily decreasing cost of electronic equipment has resulted in an increased ability to acquire these affordable and practical tools and to capitalize on their effectiveness. There is a general trend toward a paperless office environment.

WHAT IS A COMPUTER?

A computer is an electronic device operating under the control of instructions stored in its own memory unit. A computer system is a collection of devices that function together to store and process data. In a dental office a computer is a tool that helps to increase the efficiency of the business systems. A complete understanding of the manual operations of a business is an important first step toward the transition into an electronic environment. A computer is the dental office administrator's electronic aide.

Computers perform many repetitive functions with great speed and efficiency. They can, for example,

- store, process, and manipulate large amounts of data
- provide fast retrieval of information
- perform many tasks simultaneously and repetitively
- perform many complicated calculations
- produce documentation
- increase office efficiency

Fears Associated With Learning to Use Computers

Although computers can perform the tasks that previously required many manual hours, they do not replace human beings. One of the greatest fears that many people face is that human beings will eventually be replaced by machines. Computers are machines that are constructed and programmed with the intended purpose of assisting with tasks that are time-consuming and monotonous. Computers seldom make mistakes and never get bored with repetitive tasks. These machines are able to perform complicated calculations that are based on logic. However, they are not capable of generating human thought or emotion. The computer can only follow instructions and perform tasks.

Although in recent years many computer systems have become responsive to the user, some computer operators may feel a sense of loss of their own personal power to an unfeeling machine that does not provide feedback. To overcome the fear of using computers, it is helpful to view them as an organizational tool and not a threat. These instruments can provide the dental office administrator with more time for client communications and abundant marketing opportunities.

Some of the fear of learning to use computers originates from a basic fear of the unknown. Unless people clearly understand the need to convert to an electronic environment and see the ultimate benefits, they will resist learning. The fear of looking uninformed in the presence of coworkers is a major factor in the learning process. New information of any kind will be unfamiliar and cause apprehension. Once people become familiar with what they are learning, they will become more comfortable and even willing to share their knowledge.

First-time computer users may be afraid that they will break the computer, lose important information, or make irreparable mistakes. The financial investment made in computer systems can add to the fear of feeling responsible if something goes wrong. A good training program, patience, understanding, and positive reinforcement will mitigate the fears associated with learning computers and enable the dental office administrator to enter the information age with confidence.

Needs Analysis

When a dentist is considering the purchase of a computer system, he or she will often consult staff members to evaluate the needs of the practice. A computer in a dental office should be able to perform the following functions:

- perform appointment scheduling functions for multiple dental providers
- store patient records
- update patient records
- perform complex financial transactions and calculations such as account billing and reconciliation
- maintain accounts receivable and accounts payable records

- function as a reminder system for recalls
- produce daily and monthly reports
- generate insurance forms
- transmit insurance claims information (through Electronic Data Interchange)
- produce correspondence and formal written reports
- enhance marketing capabilities
- maintain clinical records

Many dental offices have computer terminals in each operatory. These allow the dentist or dental assistant to enter treatment information, schedule the next appointment, generate insurance forms, etc. That is why computer literacy or knowledge of computer concepts and applications is essential for all members of the dental team. Because training costs for personnel can account for a large portion of a computer support contract, most dentists will seek to hire someone who has previous training and experience on a dental computer system or is generally computer literate. This helps to reduce the amount of time and money required to train staff.

Hardware

A computer system consists of two major components. The first component is called the hardware. The hardware consists of the physical equipment that makes up the computer system, for example, the computer terminal, keyboard, video display terminal (or monitor), and peripheral equipment such as the printer.

Video Display Terminal

The video display terminal or monitor looks like a television screen. The monitor displays each function as it is being performed. Monitors are available in one colour (monochromatic) or in many colours (polychromatic).

Keyboard

The keyboard is the communication device that you use to instruct the computer to perform specific functions. The central portion of each keyboard is the same as a typewriter keyboard. Above the typing keys there is a set of function keys, identified as F1, F2, F3, etc. These keys perform specific functions that are written into the software program. In addition, there are special action keys that will change the function

EXHIBIT 23.1 **YOUR COMPUTER SYSTEM**

Introduction	Your ABELDent system has two major components: *hardware* and *software*. ABELDent is the primary software program.
Software	Software is the set of programmed instructions that enable the computer to accomplish the tasks specified by the operator.
ABELDent	ABELDent is the set of programs containing instructions that enable the computer to perform functions specifically for a dental office.
Hardware	Hardware is the set of physical, electronic components that comprise a computer system.
Hardware Components	The major hardware components of your system are shown below.

Computer   **Printers**

Display

System Unit   Laser

Keyboard   Dot Matrix

The Server	The server is the main computer that contains the data base for your ABELDent system. One or more "client" computers may access patient information from the server over a network cable connection. The server must operate on the Windows NT operating system while the client computers may run either Windows NT or Windows 95. The server is also the machine that is normally used to initialize the laser printer and to perform system back-ups.

Server

Client   Client

Sample provided by ABEL Computers Ltd., Burlington, Ontario.

when pressed at the same time as a function key. This means that one function key can perform several different functions. The special action keys are Ctrl (control), Alt, Shift, and Tab.

On the right side of the keyboard there are arrow keys. These are called cursor keys. A cursor is the flashing dot that identifies a specific position or field on the screen. The cursor keys may be combined with the numeric keypad that is on the right side of the keyboard. The arrows will move your cursor in the direction that is indicated. If you wish to use the numeric keypad, select Num Lock (numeric lock) and numbers will appear on the screen.

The keyboard is considered to be alphanumeric because it will communicate with the main control or central processing unit of the computer in either alphabetical or numeric format.

Mouse

You can also communicate with the computer by using a mouse pointer. A mouse is a hand-held unit that moves the on-screen pointer to allow the operator to make selections and execute commands.

Accessing functions with the mouse increases the speed and efficiency of data entry. Some computer software programs may combine mouse actions with typing shortcut keys for greater productivity.

Central Processing Unit

The central processing unit or main brain of the computer is available as a vertical tower or horizontal unit. It contains a hard drive which is a magnetic storage device to store the software programs and operating system. This is a nonremovable storage device.

TABLE 23.1 **USING A MOUSE**

ACTION	DESCRIPTION
Click	Press the left mouse button once.
Double click	Press the left mouse button quickly twice
Click and drag	Position the mouse pointer on an item. Press and hold the left mouse button to move the item to the required position. Release the mouse button.

Printer

The printer is the output device that produces printed information, referred to as hard copy. There are a variety of printers available, such as dot matrix, ink jet, and laser printers. Dot matrix printers are usually the least expensive and are particularly useful for producing multiple-copy forms. There are two types, a 9-pin and a 24-pin printer. Each one produces an image through a series of dots that are created by a number of pins pushed through a pinhead and an inked ribbon. The more pins, the higher the quality of the image that is produced.

Ink jet printers (also known as bubble jets) blow small droplets of ink through small nozzles. They produce a high-quality image and are available in colour. If the printer uses water soluble ink, however, the image may run if water is spilled on the paper. Ink jet printers produce high-quality documents quietly and quickly.

Laser printers produce an image by fusing dry toner to the paper. This process is similar to that of a photocopier. The images are produced quickly and quietly and present a nearly typeset quality. As laser printers produce optimal quality documents, they are ideally suited to produce dental insurance forms.

Modem

Information can be transmitted from one computer to another by means of a modem. The modem is a device that enables a computer or

EXHIBIT 23.2 **PRINTERS**

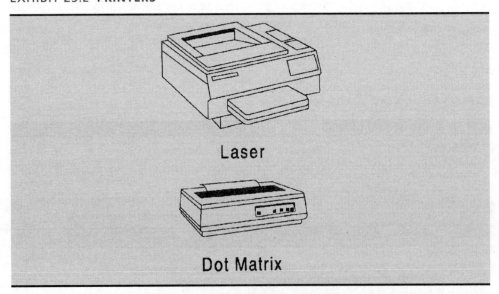

Sample provided by ABEL Computers Ltd., Burlington, Ontario.

terminal to communicate with another computer over a telephone line. This is accomplished by connecting a modem to each computer in the separate locations and then placing the phone jack into each modem. A communication software package then enables the modem to convert signals from analog devices (such as a telephone system) to digital code (that the computer understands).

Removable Disk Drive

The removable floppy disk drives are located on the front of the central processing unit. Floppy disks are removable data disks that are available in 5.25- or 3.5-inch sizes. The 5.25-inch diskettes are quickly becoming obsolete as the 3.5-inch diskettes can hold much more data than the larger disks and their hard protective shells are more durable than the "floppy" type. They store information on a magnetic medium that is contained inside the protective cover. Information can be stored on both sides of the magnetic medium; that is why they are called double-sided. Tiny electromagnetic reading heads that are located in the removable disk drive are able to read information that is stored on both sides of the disk. The data is stored within a series of small concentric tracks that are metallic particles embedded in the disk's coating.

The density of the removable diskette refers to the amount of information that can be stored on it, which is measured in bytes of information. Double-sided, high density, 3.5-inch diskettes usually store 1.44 megabytes of information. Diskettes are usually preformatted, which means that the tracks have been prepared to receive and store data.

Software

A computer follows instructions that are written by a person known as a programmer. The program instructions control the operation of the computer by processing data. The computer executes the instructions. Examples of software programs are ABELDent, WordPerfect, and Lotus 123. A dental software program has the ability to understand and perform functions that are relevant to a dental office, such as

- scheduling appointments
- entering treatment information into a patient's chart
- entering fees
- maintaining clinical information

Customized software programs can be independently written for each practice or purchased through a computer company that specializes in dental hardware and software.

PATIENT INFORMATION

A computer system will allow the dental office administrator to organize and store patient information for fast retrieval. Patient information is separated into categories and stored in the computer to provide for random access to it as needed.

Patient information should be updated every time a patient visits the dental office.

Operating Systems

A computer operating system controls the operations of the computer and the software. The operating system tells the computer how to perform functions such as loading, storing, and executing an application program. It also tells the computer how to transfer data between the input/output devices and main memory. The operating system is sometimes referred to as the computer's environment.

TABLE 23.2 PATIENT INFORMATION CATEGORIES

CATEGORY	DESCRIPTION
Personal	Demographic information
Health	Medical history
Insurance	Personal insurance plan
Treatment	Dental services completed
Treatment planning	Proposed treatment, estimates
Appointments	Detailed appointment list and recall schedule
Notes	Additional notes specific to each patient
X-rays	Mounted and dated radiographs
Imaging	Charting graphics

Some examples of operating systems are

- MS-DOS—Disk Operating System
- Windows 3.1
- Windows 95
- OS/2

In some personal computers, operators one can choose which operating system they prefer to use when they turn on the computer or switch to an alternative operating system while the computer is running.

In the MS-DOS environment, the operating system will perform tasks through a series of text-based commands. Information is stored in directories and subdirectories. The keyboard is the device used to communicate the commands to the operating system. There are many different commands with varying formats.

It is difficult to remember all of the commands, switches, and special action keys that perform functions in a DOS environment. Often a Windows environment is preferred for dental software programs.

A Windows environment displays programs and software using graphical images, called icons, on the screen. A window is a rectangular area on the screen in which you can enter or view information. The windows appear on a background called the desktop. Windows uses a *graphical user interface* (GUI, pronounced "gooey") environment. This environment allows the user to select commands or start programs by pointing to icons using a mouse and clicking to make the selection. Window sizes can be altered by using the click and drag mouse function. Window sizes can also be maximized or minimized by clicking on the up or down arrow that is located in the top right-hand corner of the screen.

TABLE 23.3 **TYPICAL DOS COMMANDS**

DRIVE	COMMAND	SOURCE	TARGET
C:\	copy	c:*.*	a:\
Backslash indicates the root directory of the drive called "C"	the action	From the root directory of "C", all files (*.*).	The target drive and directory is the root directory of "A".

Windows will allow the operator to perform multitasking, which is the ability to run more than one software application at a time. To move a window, click and drag on the title bar to the new location and release the mouse button. When several windows are open, they may overlap one another, making it difficult to find a particular application. The Program Manager is an organizing window. To close a window, double click on the minus sign located in the upper left corner of the screen.

Windows 95 is the most recent version of the Windows operating systems. It uses familiar objects such as file folders and documents to represent the desktop on the screen. The purpose of this type of graphical interface is to make the operating system more friendly and easier to use. The start button located on the task bar allows fast access to programs, documents, and files. Users of Windows 95 should be careful to follow a proper shutdown procedure from the start button menu after closing all document files. Windows 95 has enhanced multitasking features which can be accessed quickly from the task bar. If a software application remains active, it will appear in the task bar. To close the application, click on the window and the object will disappear.

Scroll bars are vertical or horizontal bars that allow the user to scroll through the document window, displaying the contents. Dialog boxes contain a choice of selections that are available to the user. A check mark appears if a selection is active. If an option is not available, it will be faded out. After the selection has been made, the user must click on OK to send the command.

ELECTRONIC DATA INTERCHANGE

The success of Electronic Data Interchange (EDI) depends on having a software program and a modem properly set up for EDI. There are five areas in the system where information must be set up for the electronic submissions of claims. In order to use EDI, all five areas must be set up correctly. Information must be entered in

- the provider file for each provider who will submit claims electronically
- the patient information area, for each patient whose claims will be submitted using EDI
- the insurance plan file for each plan which is used by a patient whose claims are submitted electronically
- the insurance carrier file, for each carrier who accepts EDI claims

EXHIBIT 23.3 COMPUTER MENU SCREEN

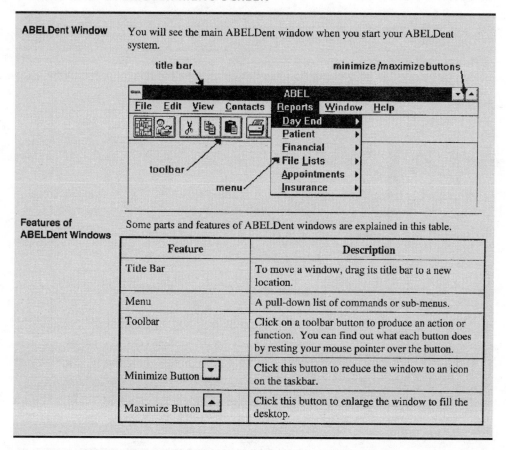

ABELDent Window

You will see the main ABELDent window when you start your ABELDent system.

Features of ABELDent Windows

Some parts and features of ABELDent windows are explained in this table.

Feature	Description
Title Bar	To move a window, drag its title bar to a new location.
Menu	A pull-down list of commands or sub-menus.
Toolbar	Click on a toolbar button to produce an action or function. You can find out what each button does by resting your mouse pointer over the button.
Minimize Button	Click this button to reduce the window to an icon on the taskbar.
Maximize Button	Click this button to enlarge the window to fill the desktop.

Sample provided by ABEL Computers Ltd., Burlington, Ontario.

ERGONOMICS

Ergonomics is the study of the design and arrangement of equipment for healthy, comfortable, safe, and efficient human interaction. Ergonomic considerations relevant to the purchase of a computer system include the following:

- a detached keyboard
- a movable screen with view angle adjustments
- high quality screen display with well-focused images
- the ability to adjust screen brightness and contrast

EXHIBIT 23.4 **EXIT STEPS**

Step	Action
1	To exit the ABELDent program, click the **Close** button ☒.
2	Exit any other programs that you are running (for example, Word, Excel, etc.) in the way suggested for those programs.
3	Click the **Start** button, and then choose **Shut Down**.
4	Click on the **Yes** button. If you forget to save changes to documents, Windows prompts you to save changes. Note: To **reboot** your computer, select the **Restart Your Computer?** option before clicking on the **Yes** button.
5	A screen message lets you know when you can safely turn off your computer.

Note: For information about the other options in the Shut Down dialog box, click the Help button.

Sample provided by ABEL Computers Ltd., Burlington, Ontario. Windows 95 is copyrighted material of Microsoft Corporation.

- a screen with antiglare coating
- screen and keyboard position at an appropriate height for the user

The user should sit directly in front of the screen in an adjustable chair with lower back support.

Care and Maintenance of Computers

Proper care and maintenance of the computer hardware and software will extend the life of the computer system and prevent unnecessary downtime. These are some basic guidelines to follow for computer maintenance:

EXHIBIT 23.5 **WINDOWS 95 INTRODUCTION**

Introducing Windows 95 ®

Introduction

The Windows 95 operating system may run on any client computer. Its graphical interface is easy to learn and is consistent from one program to another. The basic information that you will need to run ABELDent under Windows is presented here. See your *Windows 95 manual* for more information.

Basic Terms

After the initial startup, your Windows screen may look similar to the following:

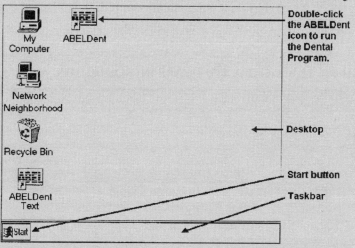

This picture illustrates some of the visual elements that make up your Windows screen. Small graphical symbols called *icons* provide quick access to application programs and utilities. At the bottom of the screen is the *taskbar*. It contains the *Start button*, which you can use to quickly start a program or to find a file. It is also the fastest way to access online help for Windows 95.

Switching Between Programs

Every time you start a program or open a window, a button representing that window appears on the taskbar. To switch between windows, just click the button for the window you want. When you close a window, its button disappears from the taskbar.

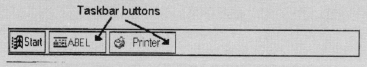

Sample provided by ABEL Computers Ltd., Burlington, Ontario. Windows 95 is copyrighted material of Microsoft Corporation.

- Shut off the power and disconnect all ports before moving the computer.
- Avoid having any liquid near the keyboard. Moisture will cause permanent damage to electronic equipment.

- Keep the keyboard covered when not in use. This helps to prevent damage from dust, staples, paper clips, etc. The keyboard is very vulnerable to damage.
- Removable diskettes are sensitive to excessive temperatures, hot and cold. Store them in a cool, dry holder.
- Do not bend, fold, or staple diskettes.
- Do not place diskettes on anything that contains a magnetic field such as the central processing unit. The diskettes store information on a magnetic medium that can become scrambled if exposed to a magnetic field.

EXHIBIT 23.6 DENTAL SOFTWARE INTRODUCTION

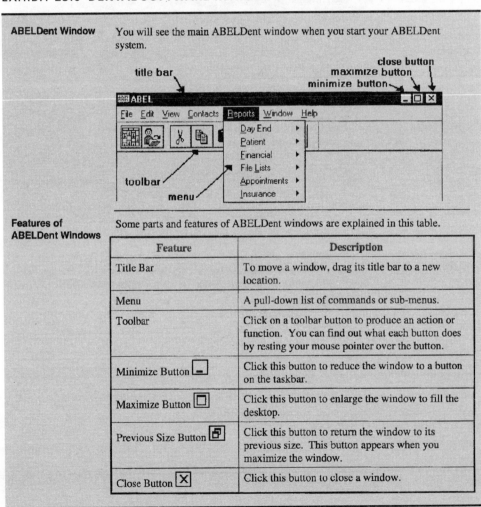

Feature	Description
Title Bar	To move a window, drag its title bar to a new location.
Menu	A pull-down list of commands or sub-menus.
Toolbar	Click on a toolbar button to produce an action or function. You can find out what each button does by resting your mouse pointer over the button.
Minimize Button	Click this button to reduce the window to a button on the taskbar.
Maximize Button	Click this button to enlarge the window to fill the desktop.
Previous Size Button	Click this button to return the window to its previous size. This button appears when you maximize the window.
Close Button	Click this button to close a window.

Sample provided by ABEL Computers Ltd., Burlington, Ontario.

EXHIBIT 23.7 **DIALOG BOX INFORMATION**

Using Dialog Boxes

Introduction

You enter most of your information into ABELDent using dialog boxes. A dialog box is a rectangular area that appears temporarily to request or supply information. For example, you might need to select certain options, type some text, or specify a setting.

Sample Dialog Box

An example of a dialog box is shown below.

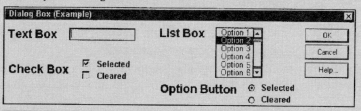

Using a Dialog Box

Dialog boxes contain different types of items. By pressing **<Tab>** you can move forward through the items on a dialog box. Pressing **<Shift + Tab>** moves backward through the items. These items include:

- Text Box. A box in which you type and edit information.
- Check box. A square box that represents an option that you can select or clear by clicking on the box or pressing the **<Space Bar>** while on this item.
- List Box. A list or pull-down list that scrolls to display available alternatives. You click on your choice using a mouse.
- Option Button. A button that allows you to pick one item from a number of exclusive options. Click on the button using the mouse to select the option. All other options will be turned off automatically.
- Command Button. A button that causes the program to take a specific action. Many dialog boxes have an **OK** button that you click when you are finished and wish to go to the next step.

Note: The ⌨ button does not work inside dialog boxes. Use the **<F1>** key to access Help. See Chapter 5 on *Finding Information Quickly* for more information.

Tab Dialog Boxes

Many information windows in ABELDent use a tabular format to help you organise and access your data. For example, patient information is separated into different categories.

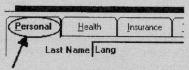

You click on a tab to display the corresponding category of information in a tab dialog box. You enter or edit information in a tab dialog box using the techniques listed in *Using a Dialog Box*.

Sample provided by ABEL Computers Ltd., Burlington, Ontario.

- Use a static mat. Computers are sensitive to static electricity. Static sprays are available and controlling the humidity is an effective way to prevent loss of data due to static. Rebooting (restarting) the computer can sometimes help to reset the system if this occurs.

EXHIBIT 23.8 EDI PROCEDURES

Patient Information	The successful submission of claims through EDI depends on the completeness and accuracy of the patient and subscriber information. Follow these steps to enter required patient information.

Step	Action
1	• See *Accessing the Patient Information Window* in online help. Once there:
2	Select the correct window and ensure that the following information is entered for a patient: • First Name • Last Name • Middle Initial (optional) • Name of school (if student = Y) • Relationship to subscriber • Sex • Birthdate
3	If the patient is a subscriber ensure that the following information is entered: • First Name • Last Name • Middle Initial (optional) • Address (including city, province) • Birthdate • Plan ID • Certificate Number • Policy Number • Division/Section Number (if required by carrier)
4.	If the patient has dual coverage, ensure that the following information is entered on the **Insurance Plans** tab dialog box: • Secondary Plan ID • Secondary Policy Number • Secondary Division/Section Number (if required by carrier) • Secondary Subscriber's Certificate Number • Relationship to Secondary Subscriber

Sample provided by ABEL Computers Ltd., Burlington, Ontario.

- Read any available computer manuals. Many support calls can be prevented if the user is willing to look up the problem in the computer manual. Each manual usually has a section on troubleshooting.
- If something appears to be wrong with the machine, do not randomly hit keys. A computer is logical and knows what the next step should be—randomly hitting keys can confuse it. If the problem is serious, call for support.

Computer Support

Most software packages have online help. However, from time to time a support call must be made to the company. Be prepared with enough information to assist the support representative in solving the problem. Often it takes a while to pinpoint the problem; however, if the representative has a clear picture of the events that preceded the breakdown, he or she is better able to offer assistance. A support contract is an agreement between the dental office and the software company to be available to assist when needed.

ASSIGNMENT

1. What is the definition of a computer?
2. What are the two main components of a computer system?
3. Describe some of the fears related to learning to use a computer system.
4. List some ergonomic recommendations to consider when working with a computer system.
5. Describe ways in which a computer can become a valuable aid to the dental office administrator.
6. Describe the functions of an operating system.
7. Define and describe GUI.

INDEX

A

Abbreviations
    charting symbols, 65
    insurance coverage, 75
    Latin, 200
    tooth surfaces, 45
ABELDent. *See also* Computers
    dialog boxes, 287
    exit steps, 284
    introduction, 276
    windows, 283, 286
Abutment, 27
Account statement, 135–37
Accounting. *See* Accounts payable,
    Accounts receivable, Banking,
    Payroll
Accounts payable, 141–50
    bill payments, 149
    cheques, 145, 147
    continuous bank balance, 147
    disbursements journal, 142, 146
    expense categories, 142–45
    inventory control, 149, 150
    petty cash fund, 147, 148
Accounts receivable, 122–40
    advance payments, 133
    aged receivables, 124
    bad debts, 133
    collection procedures, 135–39
    control account, 132
    daily balancing procedure, 131,
      132, 134
    daysheet, 130, 131
    financial arrangements, 134, 135
    leaflet receipts, 125, 127
    ledger cards, 127–30
    NSF cheques, 133, 134
    one write system, 125, 126
    refunds, 133

Acrylic restoration, 27
Action verbs, 237
Addiction, 207
Additive action, 207
Adjective, 237
Advance payments, 133
Advanced appointment system, 118,
    119
Adverb, 238
After-hours emergency callers, 107,
    108
Alphabetical filing system, 184
Alternate benefits clause, 74
Alveolar process, 40, 42, 43
Alveolar socket (alveolus), 42
Alveolectomy, 27
Amalgam, 27
Anaesthetics, 199
Angry callers, 110
Answering machine/service, 107
Antagonism, 207
Anterior teeth, 27
Antibiotics, 199, 201
Anticoagulants, 201
Anticonvulsants, 201
Antidote, 208
Antihistamines, 201
Antiselection, 70
Antrum lavage, 27
Apex, 27, 42, 43
Apical curettage, 27
Apical foramen, 42, 43
Apicoectomy, 27
Apostrophes, 245
Appliance, 27
Applied psychology, 13–18
Appointment scheduling, 86–101
    appointment book, 87, 88
    buffer zones, 96

cancellations/short notice lists, 92

changing from manual to computerized scheduling, 99

children, 97

colour coding schedules, 91, 92

confirming appointments, 89

double booking, 95

elderly patients, 97, 98

emergency vs. urgency, 95, 96

ideal day, 93, 94

nervous patients, 97

new patient procedure, 93

phone list, 90

preparing for appointments, 91, 92

scheduling appointments, 88, 89

school holidays, 97

series of appointments, 97

staff meetings, 96

Arrow keys, 277

Articulator, 27

B

Bacterial, 28

Bad debts, 133

Bank charges, 144

Bank reconciliation, 171–73

Bank statement, 171, 173

Banking, 164–74

bank statement, 171, 173

cheques, 165–68

current accounts, 165

deposits, 169, 170

reconciliation, 171–73

stop payment order, 168, 169

Barriers to communication, 22

Bi, 26

Bicuspids, 28, 40, 41

Bill payments, 149

Biopsy, 28

Birthday cards, 220, 221

Bitewing, 28

Bleaching, 28

Body gestures, 20

Bony palate, 39

Bookkeeping, 123. *See also* Accounts payable, Accounts receivable

Braces, 32

Brand named drugs, 197

Bruxism, 28

Bubble jet printers, 278

Buccal, 28

Buccal surface, 45

Buffer zones, 96

Business letters, 246–50

C

Calculus, 28

Canal, 28

Cancellations, 92

Cancelled cheque, 171

Canines, 40

Capitation program, 71, 72

Careers. *See* Job search

Caries, 28

Carious, 28

Carrier, 70

Cast metal post and core, 28

Cast space maintainer, 28

Cemento-enamel function, 42, 43

Cementum, 28, 42, 43

Cent, 26

Central processing unit, 277

Centric occlusion, 41

Cephalometric film, 28

Charting pencils, 64

Charting symbols, 63, 64

Charts. *See* Dental charts

Cheeks, 38

Chemical drug name, 197

Cheque ledger (stub), 167, 168

Cheque writer, 167

Cheques, 145, 147, 165–68

Children
    consent forms, 178
    preventive procedures, 189
    scheduling appointments, 97

Chlor/o, 27

Chronological filing system, 184,
    255, 256

Claim forms, 79–82

Clinical records. *See* Dental charts

Closed punctuation, 248

Collection agencies, 136, 139

Collection calls, 109

Collection letters, 136, 138, 139

Colons, 244

Colour coding
    appointment schedules, 91, 92
    dental charts, 64, 65
    filing system, 183, 185

Colours, 26, 27

Combination recall system, 119, 120

Combining form, 25

Commas, 241, 242

Communication skills, 18–23. *See
    also* Phraseology, Written com-
    munications

Community outreach, 218

Complete dentures, 29

Complete series radiographs, 29

Complete subject, 239

Complex sentences, 240

Composite restorations, 29

Compound sentences, 240

Computerized recall system, 120

Computerized scheduling, 99

Computers, 272–89. *See also*
    ABELDent
    care/maintenance, 284–89
    definitions, 273
    electronic data interchange, 282,
        288
    ergonomics, 283, 284

fear of learning, 273, 274
    hardware, 275–79
    needs analysis, 274, 275
    operating systems, 280–82
    patient information, 280
    software, 279, 280
    support contracts/calls, 289

Conditional responses, 16

Confidentiality
    appointment book, 87
    conversations, 63
    records, 62, 75, 76
    salary negotiations, 152

Confirming appointments, 89

Conjunction, 239

Conscious sedation, 199

Consent form, 178, 179

Consultation, 29

Continuing education, 220, 271

Continuous appointment system, 98,
    99, 118, 119

Continuous bank balance, 147

Contractions, 245

Coordinating conjunctions, 239

Coordination of benefits, 76, 78

Copayments, 72, 73

Cover letter, 264, 265

CPP deductions, 156, 158

CPT1 form, 155

Credit card payments, 169–71

Crown, 29, 43

Cumulative action, 207

Current accounts, 165

Cursor, 277

Cursor keys, 277

Cuspids, 29, 40, 41

Cyan/o, 26

D

Daily journal page, 130

Daysheet, 130, 131

Deca, 26

Deciduous teeth, 29, 42

Defence mechanisms, 18

Delegation of duties, 229, 230

Dental arch, 29, 40

Dental charts, 179–82

 charting symbols, 63, 64

 colour coding, 64, 65

 contents, 179

 corrections, 60

 ink, 60

 insurance, 75

 medical histories, 58–61

 progress notes, 181

 property ownership, 63

 purposes, 61–63

 sample chart, 66

 storage, 63

 telephone calls, and, 106

Dental disease, 189, 190, 193, 194

Dental hygienist. *See* Hygienist

Dental insurance. *See* Insurance

Dental pathology, 193, 194

Dental pulp, 29

Dental terminology, 24

 abbreviations. *See* Abbreviations

 colours, 26, 27

 glossary, 27–36

 numbers, 26

 word parts, 25

Dentin, 29, 42, 43

Dentition, 29

Deposit slip, 169, 170

Depression, 17

Diagnostic casts, 29

Dialog boxes, 282, 287

Dictionary usage, 236

Diet, 190

Disbursements journal, 142, 146

Disease, 189, 190, 193, 194

Diskettes, 279

Distal surface, 29, 44

Dont, 27

Dot matrix printers, 278

Double booking, 95, 96

Downtime, 94, 95

Drawings, 143

Drug abuse, 208

Drug action, 207, 208

Drugs. *See* Pharmacology

E

Edentulous, 30

Elderly patients, 97, 98

Electronic data interchange (EDI),
 82, 83, 282, 288

Electronic mail (e-mail), 108

Electronic marketing, 218

Emergencies, 95, 96, 105–8

Emergency relationship, 217

Employer/employee relationship, 155

Employment insurance, 156, 158

Employment opportunities, 11

Enamel, 30, 42, 43

Endocarditis, 207, 209

Endodontics, 30

Endorsement, 166

Ergonomics, 283, 284

Eruption cycle of teeth, 42–44

Erythr/o, 26

Essential clauses, 243

Exclamation mark, 241

Exclusions and/or limitations clause,
 74

Exfoliation, 43

Expense categories, 142–45

Extra-oral film, 30

F

Facial surface, 45

Facial view, 64

Fear, 16, 17, 22

Fee guide, 78, 79, 257

Felt needs, 16

Filing systems, 183–86

Financial arrangements, 134, 135
Financial records, 176, 182. *See also*
    Accounts payable, Accounts
    receivable, Banking, Payroll
Firing, 225
Fixed expenses, 143
Flossing, 192
Fluoride, 30, 191, 193
Follow-up binder, 256, 257
Follow-up calls, 110
Fractures, 30
Fragmented sentences, 240
Frenectomy, 30, 40
Frenum, 30, 39
Frequent referral program, 219
Fridge magnets, 220
Frustration, 231
Full block letter style, 248, 249

G
General anaesthetic, 199
Generic drug name, 197
Gingiva, 30, 43
Gingival papilla, 192
Gingivectomy, 30
Gingivitis, 30, 193
Gingivoplasty, 30
Glossary of dental terms, 27–36
Glossitis, 30, 194
Goals, setting, 257
Gold foil restoration, 30
Good news bulletin board, 220
Grammar, 236–39
Graphical user interface (GUI), 281
Guarantor, 70

H
Habituation, 207
Hands-free paging, 108
Hard palate, 38
Hardware, 275

Health alerts, 60, 61, 182
Health Management Organization
    (HMO), 72
Hemisection, 31
Hemostasis, 201
Heparin, 201
Hierarchy of motivational needs, 14,
    15
Hiring, 224–26
Hold button, 108
Human relations. *See* Personnel rela-
    tions
Hygienist
    continuing care appointments, 99
    employer/employee relationship,
        155
    recall appointment, 192
Hypersensitivity, 207
Hyphens, 245, 246
Hypochondria, 17
Hysteria, 17

I
Ideal day, 93, 94
Idiosyncrasy, 207
Immediate dentures, 31
Inactive records, 177
Incisal surface, 45
Incisors, 31, 40, 41
Income tax deductions, 156, 157
Indemnity contract, 71
Independent clauses, 243
Information brochures, 220
Informed consent, 178, 179
Injections, 203
Ink jet printers, 278
Inlay, 31
Inscription, 198
Insurance, 69–85
    assignment of benefits, 71
    capitation program, 71, 72

claim forms, 79–82
coordination of benefits, 76, 78
dental charts, and, 75
EDI claim submissions, 82, 83
eligibility requirements, 70, 71
exclusions and limitations, 74
group, 70
identification systems, and, 48
new patient interviews, and, 23
predetermination of benefits, 65, 75–77
preferred provider organization, 72
recalls, and, 74, 117
shared risk, 72–74
Insurance code reference sheet, 257
Insurer, 70
International Tooth Numbering System, 48–52
Interproximal, 31
Interproximal space, 44
Intolerance, 207
Intra-oral computers, 218
Intra-oral films, 31
Intramuscular injection, 203
Intravenous, 31
Introductory phrases, 243
Inventory control, 149, 150

J
Job interview, 265, 267
Job search, 258–71
attendance/punctuality, 259, 260
attitude, 260
avenues to explore, 261, 262
cover letter, 264, 265
employer concerns, 267–69
interview, 265, 267
rejection, 260, 261
résumés, 263, 264, 266
salary negotiations, 270
skills, 259
skills analysis, 262
thank-you note, 270

K
Keyboard, 275, 277
Kilo, 26

L
Labial, 31
Labial surface, 45
Laboratory fees, 143
Lactic acid, 190
Laser printers, 278
Late patients, 98
Latin abbreviations, 190
Laughing gas, 199
Leaflet receipts, 125, 127
Ledger cards, 127–30, 182
Letter styles, 246–50
Leuk/o, 27
Line of credit, 165
Lingual, 31
Lingual frenum, 39
Lingual surface, 44
Lingual view, 64
Linking verbs, 238
Lips, 38
Local anaesthesia, 31
Local anaesthetic, 199
Location, 214
Lunch hours, 88

M
Make ready area, 91
Malocclusion, 41
Mandibular, 31
Mandible, 31, 40
Marketing, 212–22
continuing education, 220
defined, 212, 213

electronic, 218
informed choices, 214, 215
location, 214
patient trust, 216, 217
product/price, 213
role of dental team, 215, 216
strategies, 217–19
suggested techniques, 219, 220
Maslow, Abraham, 14
Mastication, 31, 40
Maxilla, 40
Mediation sign-out sheet, 204
Medical histories, 58–61, 182
Medications. *See* Pharmacology
Melan/o, 26
Mesial, 31
Mesial surface, 44
Message taking, 110–12
Midline, 48
Midsagittal plane, 48
Milli, 26
Missed appointments, 92, 93
Mixed dentition, 31
Mixed dentition stage, 43
Mnemonic devices, 235
Modem, 278, 279
Modified block letter style, 248, 250
Molars, 31, 41
Mono, 26
Morning mini-meeting, 229
Morphology, 31
Motivation, 14, 15
Mouse, 277
Mouth
    parts, 38–40
    quadrants, 48–50
MS-DOS, 281

N
Narcotic, 32
Narcotics control, 204–6, 208
Necrosis, 32

Necrotic, 32
Necrotizing ulcerative gingivitis, 194
Nervous patients, 97
Neurotic behaviour, 17
New employees, 152–55
New patient interview, 23
New patient procedure, 93
New patient registration form, 178, 180
Newsletter, 219
Nitrous oxide/oxygen, 32, 199
No cavity club, 220
Nona, 26
Nonessential clauses, 243
Normal behaviour, 17
Noun, 236
NSF cheques, 133, 134, 168
Numbers, 26
Numeric keypad, 277
Numerical filing system, 184
Nutrition, 32, 190

O
Obturator, 32
Occlusal, 32
Occlusal equilibration, 32
Occlusal film, 32
Occlusal surface, 45
Occlusal view, 64
Occlusion, 41
Octa, 26
Office environment, 8, 9
Office hours, 88
Office policies, 227, 228
1 to 31 file, 256
One write bookkeeping system, 125, 126
Onlay, 32
Open punctuation, 248
Operating systems, 280–82
Oral aerosol inhalers, 203
Oral hygiene instruction, 32

Oral pathology, 32
Oral suspension, 202
Organism, 32
Organizational techniques, 253–57
Orthodontic, 32
Orthodontic services, 73
Out-guides, 184
Overbite, 32
Overdose, 208
Overhang, 32
Overview, 3–7

P
Palate, 33, 38
Pallor, 33
Palmer's identification system, 53–56
Panalypse, 33
Panoramic film, 33
Panorex, 33
Parentheses, 246
Partial denture, 33
Parts of speech, 236–39
Pathology, 193, 194
Patient attitudes toward health care, 115
Patient behaviour, 15–18
Patient education, 188, 189. *See also* Oral hygiene instruction
Patient trust, 216, 217
Patient's right to privacy. *See* Confidentiality
Pavlov, Ivan, 16
Payee, 166
Payer, 145
Payment options, 135, 169–71
Payroll, 151–63
    employer/employee relationship, 155
    information, sources of, 152, 161
    new employees, 152–55
    record of employment, 161
    record retention, 152

source deductions, 155–60
T4 slips, 160, 162, 163
time records, 152
vacation pay, 160
PD7A remittance form, 158–60
Pendulous palate, 39
Penicillin, 201, 207
Periapical radiograph, 33
Period, 241
Periodontal disease, 33
Periodontal ligament, 42
Periodontitis, 193, 194
Permanent dentition, 33
Personal calls, 109
Personal grooming/mannerisms, 230, 231
Personal pronoun, 237
Personal qualities, 9–11
Personnel relations, 223–33
    delegation of duties, 229, 230
    dress/mannerisms/behaviour, 230, 231
    firing, 225
    hiring, 224–26
    morning mini-meetings, 229
    office policies, 227, 228
    problem solving, 231, 232
    résumés, 227
    staff incentives, 232, 233
    staff meetings, 228
Petty cash fund, 147, 148
Pharmacology, 33, 196–211
    drug action, 207, 208
    medications management, 208
    methods of administering drugs, 202, 203
    narcotics control, 204–6
    premedication procedures, 208–10
    prescription drugs, 196–202
Philtrum, 40
Phobia, 17
Phraseology

angry callers, 110
   positive communications, 21
   telephone conversations, 104
Physiology, 33
Pit and fissure sealants, 33, 189
Plaque, 33, 190
Pocket toothbrush, 219
Pontic, 33
Posterior teeth, 33
Predeterminations, 65, 75–77, 256, 257
Predicate, 240
Preferred Provider Organization (PPO), 72
Prefix, 25
Premedication procedures, 208–10
Premolar, 33
Prepaid insurance program, 71
Preposition, 238, 239
Prescription, 197–99
Preventive dentistry, 187–89
Price, 213
Primary, 34
Primary dentition, 43, 51
Printers, 278
Private contractors, 155
Problem solving techniques, 231, 232
Procedure codes, 79, 80
Procedures and protocol manual, 253–55
Professional associations, 271
Program Manager, 282
Programmer, 279
Pronoun, 236
Proof of posting, 131
Prophy-jet, 192
Prophylactic antibiotics, 208
Prophylaxis, 34, 192
Protecting patients, 9
Proximal surfaces, 44

Psychotic behaviour, 17
Pulp, 34, 42, 43
Pulp chamber, 29
Pulpectomy, 34
Pulpotomy, 34
Punctuation, 241–46
Purging charts, 177

Q
Quad, 26
Question mark, 241
Quint, 26
Quotation marks, 244, 245

R
Radiographs, 34, 76
Radiology, 34
Rear delivery systems, 9
Recall appointment, 192, 193
Recall systems, 114–21
   combination system, 119, 120
   computerized system, 120
   continuous appointment system, 98, 99, 118, 119
   hints/tips, 98, 99, 114–16
   insurance, and, 74
   mail system, 117, 118
   telephone system, 109, 110, 116, 117
Receiver General remittances, 143, 153–60
Reception area, 8, 9
Receptor, 207
Record of employment, 161
Records management, 175–86
   clinical records, 178–82. *See also* Dental charts
   confidentiality, 175–76
   filing systems, 183–86
   financial records, 176, 182
   inactive records, 177

informed consent, 178, 179
    protection of records, 176, 177
    purging charts, 177
    release of information, 178
    retention of records, 152, 177
Red, 60
Refill information, 198
Registration form, 178, 180
Relative pronoun, 237
Release of information, 178
Reline, 34
Removable disk drive, 279
Respondeat superior, 62
Responsive listening, 20
Restorative/remedial relationship,
    217
Restrictive endorsement, 166, 167
Résumés, 227, 263, 264, 266
Retention of records, 152, 177
Retentive pins, 34
Revolving credit, 165
Root canal therapy, 34
Root canals, 42, 43

S
Salaries, 143, 151, 152
Salary negotiations, 152, 270
Scaling, 34
School holidays, 97, 110
Screening calls, 112, 113
Scroll bars, 282
Sealants application, 189
Sedation, 34
Sedatives, 202
Selection of dental office, 7, 8
Self-addressed postcard, 99, 119
Self-care relationship, 217
Semicolons, 243, 244
Sentence structure, 239
Sept, 26
Server, 276

Sext, 26
Shedding, 43
Short notice list, 92
Side effect, 202, 207
Signature, 198
Silicate restoration, 34
Simple sentences, 240
Simple subject, 239
Smile, 115, 188
Smile makeover, 219
SOAP, 62
Social insurance number (SIN), 153,
    155
Socket, 34
Soft palate, 39
Software, 279, 280
Source deductions, 152, 155–60
Special occasion prophylaxis, 219
Spell checker, 249, 250
Spelling, 235, 236
Splinting, 34
Spoken words. *See* Phraseology
Staff incentives, 232, 233
Staff meetings, 96, 228
Stainless steel crown, 34
Static mat, 288
Stimulants, 202
Stock solution, 202
Stop payment order, 168, 169
Subcutaneous injection, 203
Subject, 239
Sublingual, 35
Subscriber, 70
Subscription, 198
Suffix, 25
Sulcus, 35, 192
Sunglasses, 9
Superscription, 198
Support contract, 289
Suppositories, 203
Surgery, 35

Syncope, 35
Syndrome, 35
Synergism, 207
Systems relationship, 217

T

T4 slips, 160, 162, 163
Tartar, 35, 190
Task priority list, 255
Tax deductions tables, 156, 157
TD1 form, 152–54
Teeth
    eruption cycle, 42–44
    identification/numbering systems.
      See Tooth identification/number-
      ing systems
    structure, 42, 43
    surfaces, 44, 45
    types, 40, 41
    views, 64
Telephone usage, 102–13
    after-hours emergency calls, 107,
      108
    angry callers, 110
    answering machine/service, 107
    closure, 105
    collection calls, 109
    continuing care calls, 109, 110,
      116, 117
    emergency vs. urgency, 105–7
    equipment/technology, 106–8
    follow-up calls, 110
    gathering information, 105
    greeting, 105
    hands-free paging, 108
    hold button, 108
    legal issues, 106
    message taking, 110–12
    personal calls, 109
    phraseology, 104
    screening calls, 112, 113

    time management, 108, 109
    voice mail, 108
    voice quality, 103, 104
Temporomandibular joint (TMJ), 35,
    40
Terminology. *See* Dental terminology
Time management, 98, 99
Time records, 152
Time unit (TU), 87
Tissue, 35
Tolerance, 207
Tongue, 39
Tooth decay, 189, 190
Tooth identification/numbering
    systems
    importance, 47, 48
    international tooth numbering
      system, 48–52
    Palmer's identification system,
      53–56
    universal tooth numbering system,
      52, 53
Toothbrushing, 191, 192
Torus, 35
Toxic, 35
Tranquilizers, 35, 202
Transdermal patches, 203
Transferring patient records, 63
Transverse plane, 49
Treatment, levels of, 62
Trench mouth, 194
Tri, 26
Two-digit numbering system, 48–52

U

Uni, 26
Universal Tooth Numbering System,
    52, 53
Urgency vs. emergency, 95, 96,
    105–7

Uvula, 39

V

Vacation pay, 160, 161
Values, 16
Variable expenses, 143
Vasoconstrictors, 201
Vasodilators, 201
Verb, 237, 238
Vestibular, 35
Vestibular surfaces, 39, 45
Vestibule, 35, 39
Video display terminal, 275, 276
Vitality test, 35
Voice mail, 108
Voided cheque, 167

W

Wellness days, 233
Windows, 281, 282
Windows 95, 282, 285
Wisdow teeth, 41, 44

Word parts, 25
Wound, 36
Written communications, 234–52
    clarity, 235
    conciseness, 235
    dictionary usage, 236
    grammar, 236–39
    letter styles, 246–50
    punctuation, 241–46
    sentence structure, 239–41
    spelling, 235, 236
Wrongful dismissal, 225
Wrongful hiring, 224

X

X-ray, 36. *See also* Radiograph
X-ray procedures, 9
Xanth/o, 27
Xanthodont, 27

Z

Zinc oxide and eugenol (ZOE), 36

A COMMUNITY OF LEARNING SOLUTIONS

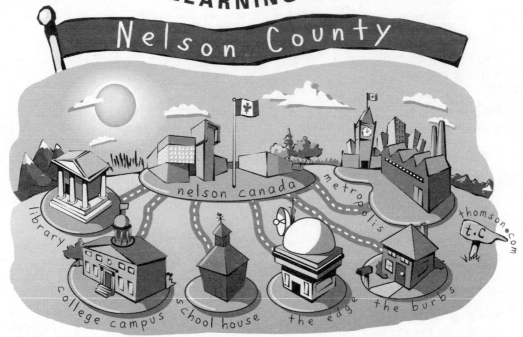

Nelson County

library · nelson canada · metropolis · thomson.com · t.c · college campus · school house · the edge · the burbs

Visit us on the Web at **http://www.nelson.com**

To the owner of this book

We hope that you have enjoyed *The Canadian Dental Office Administrator,* and
we would like to know as much about your experiences with this text as you
would care to offer. Only through your comments and those of others can we
learn how to make this a better text for future readers.

School _____ Your instructor's name _____

Course _____ Was the text required? _____ Recommended? _____

1. What did you like the most about *The Canadian Dental Office Administrator?*
   _____
   _____
   _____

2. How useful was this text for your course?
   _____
   _____
   _____

3. Do you have any recommendations for ways to improve the next edition of
   this text?
   _____
   _____
   _____

4. In the space below or in a separate letter, please write any other comments
   you have about the book. (For example, please feel free to comment on
   reading level, writing style, terminology, design features, and learning aids.)
   _____
   _____
   _____

Optional

Your name _____ Date _____

May ITP Nelson quote you, either in promotion for *The Canadian Dental Office
Administrator* or in future publishing ventures?

Yes _____ No _____

Thanks!

PLEASE TAPE SHUT. DO NOT STAPLE.

TAPE SHUT

TAPE SHUT

- - - FOLD HERE - - -

 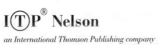 **I(T)P® Nelson**
an International Thomson Publishing company

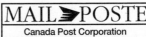
MAIL⟩POSTE
Canada Post Corporation
Société canadienne des postes

Postage paid	Port payé
if mailed in Canada	si posté au Canada
Business Reply	Réponse d'affairess

0066102399   **01**

TAPE SHUT

TAPE SHUT

0066102399-M1K5G4-BR01

ITP NELSON
MARKET AND PRODUCT DEVELOPMENT
P.O. BOX 60223 STN BRN 8
TORONTO ON M7Y 2H1

123081